An Index of Medicinal Herbs and Their Uses

By

Harold Ward

British Library Cataloguing-in-Publication Data
A catalogue record for this book is available from
the British Library

A Short History of Herbalism

Herbalism ('herbology' or 'herbal medicine') is the use of plants for medicinal purposes, and the study of such use. It covers all sorts of medicinal plants, natural remedies or cures, traditional and alternative medicines. Modern medicine tends to categorise herbalism firmly as an 'alternative therapy' as its practice is not strictly based on evidence gathered using the scientific method. Modern medicine does make use of many plant-derived compounds however, as the basis for evidence-tested pharmaceutical drugs. *Phytotherapy* also works to apply modern standards of effectiveness testing to medicines derived from natural sources.

Medicinal plants have been identified and used throughout human history. Archaeological evidence indicates that the use of medicinal plants dates at least to the Paleolithic age, approximately 60,000 years ago. Written evidence of herbal remedies dates back over 5,000 years to the Sumeranians, who created long lists of useful plants. A number of ancient cultures wrote on plants and their medical uses. In ancient Egypt, herbs are mentioned in Egyptian medical papyri, depicted in tomb illustrations, or on rare occasions found in medical jars containing trace amounts of herbs. The earliest known Greek 'herbals' were those of Diocles of Carystus, written during the third century BC, and one by Krateuas from the first century BC. Only a few fragments of these works have survived intact, but from what remains scholars have noted that there is a large amount of overlap with the Egyptian herbals.

Seeds likely used for herbalism have been found in archaeological sites of Bronze Age China dating from the Shang Dynasty, and herbs were also common in the medicine of ancient India, where the principal treatment for diseases was diet. *De Materia Medica* (an encyclopaedia and pharmacopoeia of herbs and medicines), written between 50 and 70 AD by a Roman physician, Pedanius Dioscorides, is a particularly important example of such writings; focused on the diet and 'natural remedies.' The documentation of herbs and their uses was a central part of both Western and Eastern medical scholarship through to the eighteenth century, and these works played an important role in the development of the science of botany too. Dandelion for instance, was used as an effective laxative and diuretic, and as a treatment for bile or liver problems, whilst the essential oil of common thyme was (and is) utilised as a powerful antiseptic and antifungal. Before the advent of modern antibiotics, oil of thyme was additionally used to medicate bandages.

The fifteenth, sixteenth and seventeenth centuries were the great ages of herbal remedies; with many corresponding texts being published. The first 'Herbal' to be published in English was the anonymous *Grete Herball* of 1526. The two best-known herbals in English were *The Herball or General History of Plants* (1597) by John Gerard and *The English Physician Enlarged* (1653) by Nicholas Culpeper. Culpeper's blend of traditional medicine with astrology, magic and folklore was ridiculed by the physicians of his day, yet his book - like Gerard's and other herbals, enjoyed phenomenal popularity. Natural medicines gradually waned in popularity as the 1900s progressed however, and the twentieth century also saw the slow erosion of plants as the pre-eminent sources of therapeutic effects.

Despite this, today the World Health Organization (WHO) estimates that eighty percent of the population of some Asian and African countries use herbal medicine for some aspect of primary health care. Pharmaceuticals are prohibitively expensive for most of the world's inhabitants, half of which lives on less than two American dollars a day. In comparison, herbal medicines can be grown from seed or gathered from nature at little or no cost. In actual fact, many of the pharmaceuticals currently available to physicians have a long history of use as herbal remedies, including opium, aspirin, digitalis and quinine. As is evident from this incredibly short history of herbalism and natural plant remedies – it is an aspect of human medicine with an incredibly long, varied and intriguing record. With many such traditional cures still used in the present; the multifaceted uses of plants continues to surprise us. We hope the reader enjoys this book.

MEDICINAL AND OTHER HERBS

ADONIS. *Adonis vernalis.* N.O. *Ranunculaceæ.*

Synonym : False Hellebore, Pheasant's Eye.
Habitat : Cornfields and meadows.
Features : Stem up to one foot high. Leaves alternate, divided pinnately into linear segments. Flowers large, yellow, solitary at termination of stem. Oval head of achenes succeeds flower.
Part used : Herb.
Action : Cardiac, tonic, diuretic.

Highly esteemed in cases where stimulation of heart's action is necessary, heart strain and cardiac dropsy. Diuretic qualities of value in kidney affections. Dose, 1-2 drops of the fluid extract.

AGRIMONY. *Agrimonia eupatoria.* N.O. *Rosaceæ.*

Synonym : Stickwort.
Habitat : Hedgerows, field borders and dry waste places.
Features : One of our prettiest wild plants, the erect, round, hairy stem reaching a height of two feet. The numerous pinnate leaves, hairy on both sides, and 5-6 inches long, grow alternately, having 3-5 pairs of lanceolate, toothed leaflets, with intermediate smaller ones, and still smaller ones between these. The many small, star-like, bright yellow flowers are arranged in long, tapering spikes. The root is woody, and the seeds form little burs, the taste being astringent and slightly bitter.
Part used : The whole herb.
Action : Acts as a mild astringent, tonic and diuretic, these qualities being useful in loose coughs and relaxed bowels.

Agrimony is an old remedy for debility, as it gives tone to the whole system. It is administered as a decoction of one ounce to 1½ pints water, simmered down to 1 pint, in half teacupful or larger doses, and may be sweetened with honey or black treacle if desired. The herb has been recommended for dyspepsia, but is probably only useful in this disorder when carefully combined with other more directly operating agents.

ANGELICA. *Angelica archangelica.* N.O. *Umbelliferæ.*

Synonym : Garden Angelica.

Habitat : Marshes and watery places generally.

Features : Stem up to five feet high ; erect, shiny, striated. Leaves lanceolate, serrate, terminal leaflet lobed. Umbels globular. Root fleshy, aromatic, much branched below.

Part used : Root, herb, seed.

Action : Carminative, stimulant, expectorant, diaphoretic, diuretic.

Infusion of 1 ounce herb to 1 pint boiling water. Dose, a wineglassful frequently. Used in coughs, colds, urinary disorders. The sweetmeat known as candied angelica is made by preserving the dried leaf stalks with sugar.

AVENS. *Geum urbanum.* N.O. *Rosaceæ.*

Synonym : Colewort, Herb Bennet.

Habitat : Hedges, woods and shady banks.

Features : This slender, sparsely branched plant reaches a height of one to two feet. The stem leaves have two leaflets, with one margin-toothed terminal lobe. The root leaves are on long stalks with two small leaflets at the base. The yellow, erect flowers, with naked styles, appear between May and September. The root is short, hard and rough, with light brown rootlets.

Part used : Herb and root.

Action : Astringent, tonic, antiseptic and stomachic.

The properties of Avens make for success in the treatment of diarrhœa and dysentery. The tonic effect upon the glands of the stomach and alimentary tract point to its helpfulness in dyspepsia. In general debility continued use has had good results. The astringent qualities may also be utilized in cases of relaxed throat. Although wineglassful doses three or four times daily of the 1 ounce to 1 pint infusion are usually prescribed, Avens may be taken freely, and is, indeed, used by country people in certain districts as a beverage in place of tea or coffee.

BALM. *Melissa officinalis.* N.O. *Labiatæ.*

Synonym : Lemon Balm, Sweet Balm.

Habitat : Borders of woods and in hedges, particularly in south of England. Common in gardens.

Features : Stem one to two feet high, freely branched, square, smoothish. Leaves stalked, opposite, broadly ovate, coarsely serrate, wrinkled, hairy. Numerous small, white or yellowish flowers, in loose bunches from leaf axils. Roots long, slender, creeping. Taste and odour of lemon.

Part used : Herb.

Action : Carminative, diaphoretic, tonic.

In influenza and feverish colds, to induce perspiration. Aids digestion. Infusion of 1 ounce to 1 pint boiling water, taken freely.

BALMONY. *Chelone glabra.* N.O. *Scrophulariaceæ.*

Synonym : Bitter Herb, Snake Head, Turtle Bloom, Turtle Head·

Habitat : Common in North America.

Features : Short-stalked leaves, opposite, oblong, lanceolate. Fruits ovate, half-inch long, bunched on short spike, two-celled, with roundish, winged, dark-centred seeds. Very bitter taste.

Part used : Leaves.

Action : Anthelmintic, detergent, tonic.

Used in constipation, dyspepsia, debility, and children's worms. Sometimes added to alteratives. Infusion of 1 ounce to 1 pint water in wineglassful doses. Powdered herb, 5-10 grains.

BARBERRY. *Berberis vulgaris.* N.O. *Berberidaceæ.*

Synonym : Berberidis, Berbery, Gouan.

Habitat : Woods and hedges, also gardens.

Features : Shrub or bush, three to eight feet high. Leaves obovate, bristly serratures. Flowers bright yellow clusters, raceme, pendulous. Berries red, oblong. Stem bark thin, yellowish-grey externally, inner surface orange yellow, separating in layers. Root dark brown, short fracture. Very bitter taste.

Part used : Bark, rootbark.

Action : Tonic, antiseptic, purgative.

Jaundice and other liver derangements. General debility. Regulates digestion, corrects constipation. ¼ teaspoonful of powdered bark, three or four times daily.

BAYBERRY. *Myrica cerifera.* N.O. *Myricaceæ.*

Synonym : Candleberry, Waxberry, Wax Myrtle.

Habitat : Near the sea in pastures and on stony soils.

Features : The bark has a white, peeling epidermis covering a hard, reddish-brown layer beneath. It is slightly fibrous on the inner surface, and the fracture is granular. The taste is pungent, astringent and bitter, the odour faintly aromatic.

Part used : The bark is the only part of the Bayberry shrub now used as a medicine.

Action : A powerful stimulant, astringent and tonic to the alimentary tract.

Bayberry bark is one of the most widely used agents in the herbal practice. It figures in many of the compound powders and is the base of the celebrated composition powder, a prescription of which will be found in the "Herbal Formulæ" section of this volume. In cases of coldness of the extremities, chills and influenza, an infusion of 1 ounce of the powdered bark to 1 pint of water is taken warm. This assists circulation and promotes perspiration, especially when combined with Cayenne as in the formula referred to above. As an antiseptic the powder is added to poultices for application to ulcers, sores and wounds. It also makes an excellent snuff for nasal catarrh, and an ingredient in tooth powders, for which a prescription is given in the section previously mentioned.

The virtues of Bayberry bark were recognized and used beneficially by the herbalists of many generations ago. Indeed, their enthusiasm for this, as for certain other remedies also extremely efficacious within proper limits, led them to ascribe properties to the bark which it does not possess. Many affections of the uterine system, fistula, and even cancer were said to yield to its influence.

Even in these cases, however, Bayberry bark certainly did less harm than many of the methods employed by the more orthodox practitioners of that time!

BISTORT. *Polygonum bistorta.* N.O. *Polygonaceæ.*

Synonym : Adderwort, Patient Dock, Snakeweed.

Habitat : Found growing in damp meadows in many parts of Britain, and is also distributed throughout Northern Europe, as well as Northern and Western Asia.

Features : The oval leaves, similar in appearance to those of the Dock, are blue-green above, grey and purplish underneath, and spring from the roots. The leaf stalks and blades are six to eight inches long, the slender flower stems carrying fewer and smaller leaves, reaching to a height of from one to two feet. A dense, cylindrical spike of pale-hued flowers blossoms from the top of the stem between June and September.

Part used : The root is the part in most demand, and is reddish-brown in colour.

Action : There is no odour, and the taste is astringent, which is the chief therapeutic action of the root—indeed it is, perhaps, the most powerful astringent in the botanic practice.

5

The decoction of 1 ounce of the crushed root to 1 pint (reduced) of water is used chiefly in hemorrhages and as a gargle and mouth-wash in cases of sore throat or gums. Combined with Flag-root it has been known to give relief from intermittent fever and ague. The old-time herbalists enthused over the virtues of Bistort root in "burstings, bruises, falls, blows and jaundice."

BITTER ROOT. *Apocynum androsæmifolium.* N.O. *Asclepiadaceæ.*

Synonym : Dogsbane, Milkweed.

Habitat : Indigenous to North America.

Features : Root is nearly three-quarters of an inch thick, light brown, transversely-wrinkled bark, easily parting from white, woody centre ; groups of stone cells in outer bark. Whole plant gives a gelatinous, milky juice when wounded.

Part used : Root.

Action : Cathartic, diuretic, detergent, emetic, tonic.

2-5 grains thrice daily as a general tonic, useful in dyspepsia. 5-15 grain doses in cardiac dropsy. Has been recommended in the treatment of Bright's disease. Large doses cause vomiting. Tendency to gripe can be eliminated by adding Peppermint, Calamus or other carminative.

BLACK HAW. *Viburnum prunifolium.* N.O. *Caprifoliaceæ.*

Synonym : American Sloe, Stagbush.

Habitat : Dry woods, throughout Central and Southern States of North America.

Features : A tree-like shrub, ten to twenty feet high. Fruit shiny black, sweet and edible. Young bark glossy purplish-brown, with scattered warts. Old bark greyish-brown, inner surface white. Fracture short. Root bark cinnamon colour. Taste bitter, astringent.

Part used : Root bark (preferred) ; also bark of stem and branches.

Action : Uterine tonic, nervine, anti-spasmodic.

Uterine weaknesses, leucorrhœa, dysmenorrhœa. Prevention of miscarriage—given four or five weeks before. Infusion of 1 ounce to 1 pint of boiling water—tablespoonful doses.

BLOOD ROOT. *Sanguinaria canadensis.* N.O. *Papaveraceæ.*

Habitat : Widely distributed throughout North America.

Features : Root reddish-brown, wrinkled lengthwise, about half-inch thick. Fracture short. Section whitish, with many small, red resin cells which sometimes suffuse the whole. Heavy odour, bitter and harsh to the taste.

Part used : Root.

Action : Stimulant, tonic, expectorant.

Pulmonary complaints and bronchitis. Should be administered in whooping-cough and croup until emesis occurs. The powdered root is used as a snuff in nasal catarrh, and externally in ringworm and other skin eruptions. The American Thomsonians use it in the treatment of adenoids. Dose, 10 to 20 grains of the powdered root.

BLUE FLAG. *Iris versicolor.* N.O. *Iridaceæ.*

Synonym : Flag Lily, Liver Lily, Snake Lily, Water Lily.

Habitat : Marshy places in Central America.

Features : Rhizome cylindrical, compressed towards larger end, where is cup-shaped stem scar. Breaks with sharp fracture, showing dark purple internally. Taste, acrid and pungent.

Part used : Root.

Action : Alterative, diuretic, cathartic.

Skin affections ; stimulates liver and other glands. Dose of the powdered root, 20 grains as a cathartic.

c—h

BLUE MALLOW. *Malva sylvestris.* N.O. *Malvaceæ.*

Synonym : Cheese Flower, Common Mallow, Mauls.

Habitat : Around hedges and roadsides.

Features : Several erect, hairy stems, two to three feet high. Leaf and flower stalks also hairy. Roundish leaf has five to seven lobes, middle one longest. Numerous flowers (June-September), large reddish-purple, clustered four or five together on axillary stalk.

Part used : Flowers, herb.

Action : Demulcent, mucilaginous, pectoral.

1 ounce to 1 pint infusion makes a popular cough and cold remedy.

BONESET. *Eupatorium perfoliatum.* N.O. *Compositæ.*

Synonym : Indian Sage, Thoroughwort.

Habitat : Damp places.

Features : One or more erect stems, branched at top. Leaves opposite, lanceolate, four to six inches long, united at base, crenate edges, tiny, yellow resin dots beneath. Flowers August to October. Persistently bitter taste.

Part used : Herb.

Action : Diaphoretic, febrifuge, tonic, laxative, expectorant.

Influenza and feverish conditions generally, for which purpose it is very successfully used by the American negroes. Also used in catarrhs. The infusion of 1 ounce to 1 pint boiling water may be given in wineglassful doses frequently, hot as a diaphoretic and febrifuge, cold as a tonic.

F. H. England, of the College of Medicine and Surgery, Chicago (Physio-Medical) says : "It is a pure relaxant to the liver. It acts slowly and persistently. Its greatest power is manifested upon the stomach, liver, bowels and uterus."

BROOM. *Cytisus scoparius.* N.O. *Leguminosæ.*

Synonym : Irish Broom and Besom.

Habitat : Dry, hilly wastes.

Features : The stem is angular, five-sided, dark green, and branches at an acute angle. Yellow pea-like flowers appear in May and June. The lower leaves are on short stalks and consist of three small obovate leaflets, the upper leaves being stalkless and frequently single.

Part used : Tops.

Action : Powerfully diuretic.

Broom tops are often used with Agrimony and Dandelion root for dropsy and liver disorders. For this purpose a decoction of 1 ounce each of Broom tops and Agrimony and ½ ounce Dandelion root to 3 pints of water simmered down to 1 quart is taken in wineglassful doses every four or five hours.

Coffin recommends us to : "Take of broom-tops, juniper-berries and dandelion-roots, each half-an-ounce, water, a pint and a half, boil down to a pint, strain, and add half-a-teaspoonsful of cayenne pepper. Dose, half-a-wineglassful four times a day."

BRYONY. *Bryonia alba.* N.O. *Cucurbitaceæ.*

Synonym : Bryonia, English Mandrake, Mandragora, Wild Vine.

Habitat : Hedges and thickets.

Features : Stem rough, hairy, freely branched, climbs several feet by numerous curling tendrils. Leaves vine-like, five- or seven-lobed, coarse and rough. Flowers (May to September), white, green-veined, in axillar panicles. Berries scarlet when ripe. Branched root one to two feet long, white internally and externally. Not to be confused with American Mandrake (q.v.).

Part used : Root.

Action : Cathartic, hydragogue.

Cough, influenza, bronchitis. Cardiac disorders resulting from rheumatism and gout. Is also used in malarial and zymotic diseases. Dose of the fluid extract, $\frac{1}{2}$ to 1 drachm. Large doses to be avoided.

BUCHU. *Barosma betulina.* N.O. *Rutaceæ.*

Habitat : South Africa, from where the leaves are imported.

Features : Three varieties of Buchu leaves are used therapeutically : (1) *Barosma betulina* or Round Buchu are rhomboid-obovate in form with blunt, recurved apex, and are preferred to either (2) *Barosma crenulata* or oval Buchu, the apex of which leaf is *not* recurved ; or (3) *Barosma serratifolia* or long Buchu, named from its distinctive, serrate-edged leaf and truncate apex.

Part used : Leaves.

Action : Diuretic, diaphoretic, stimulant.

Complaints of the urinary system, especially gravel and inflammation or catarrh of the bladder. Infusion of 1 ounce leaves to 1 pint water three or four times daily in wineglass doses.

BUCKBEAN. *Menyanthes trifoliata.* N.O. *Gentianaceæ.*

Synonym : Bogbean, Marsh or Water Trefoil.

Habitat : Low-lying, marshy lands.

Features : Stem and stalk soft and pithy. Thin, brittle, dark green leaves with long stalks and three obovate leaflets, about two inches long by one inch broad, entire edges. Very bitter taste.

Part used : Herb.

Action : Tonic, deobstruent.

Of special use as a bitter tonic ; with suitable alteratives, etc., in rheumatism and skin diseases. Frequent wineglass doses of the 1 ounce to 1 pint infusion. Coffin recommends for dyspepsia.

BUGLEWEED. *Lycopus virginicus*. N.O. *Labiatæ*.

Synonym : Sweet Bugle, Water Bugle.

Habitat : Shady and damp places in the northern regions of U.S.A.

Features : Stem smooth, square, up to eighteen inches high. Leaves opposite, short-stalked, elliptic-lanceolate, serrate above, entire lower down. Small white flowers, in axillary clusters. Bitter taste.

Part used : Herb.

Action : Sedative, astringent.

Coughs, pulmonary hemorrhage. Dose, frequent wineglasses of the 1 ounce to 1 pint infusion. England says, "Lycopus and Capsicum is *the* remedy for hemorrhage from the lungs."

BUGLOSS. *Echium vulgare*. N.O. *Boraginaceæ*.

Synonym : Blueweed, Viper's Bugloss.

Habitat : Rubbish heaps and waste land, particularly in chalky districts.

Features : Many stems grow from root to a height of two feet, prickly and hairy. Root leaves stalked, stem leaves sessile, both narrow and tapering. Flowers, five-petalled, bright red, rapidly changing to deep blue, irregularly tubular, funnel-shaped, stamens reaching beyond mouth of flower, clustered on short curved spikes growing from side of stem.

Part used : Herb.

Action : Demulcent, expectorant, diaphoretic.

Two to four tablespoonful doses of the 1 ounce to 1 pint infusion are given for the reduction of feverish colds and in inflammatory conditions of the respiratory tract.

BURDOCK. *Arctium lappa.* N.O. *Compositæ.*

Synonym : Hill, Lappa, Thorny Burr.

Habitat : This large plant, which grows to a height of five feet, is very commonly met along roadsides and in all waste places—indeed, wherever we see nettles, there also will be found Burdock.

Features : Stout stems with wide spreading branches carrying alternately fleshy, heart-shaped leaves. The purple flowers bloom luxuriously in July and August, and the bristly burs or bracts adhere lightly to the clothes and coats of animals. The root is thick, brownish-grey externally, whitish inside. Roots and seeds have a sweetish, slimy taste, the leaves and stems being bitter.

Part used : Root, seeds and the herb itself are used.

Action : Possesses alterative, diuretic and diaphoretic qualities, the root and herb being predominantly alterative, while the seeds affect more specifically the kidneys.

The liquid from 1 ounce of the root boiled in 1½ pints of water simmered down to 1 pint, is taken four times daily in wineglass doses for many forms of skin trouble, noticeably boils, carbuncles and similar eruptions. Obstinate cases of eczema and even psoriasis have been known to yield to these decoctions of Burdock root, either alone or combined with other remedies.

An excellent lotion may be made by infusing the leaves in the proportion of 1 ounce to 1 pint of water.

BURR MARIGOLD. *Bidens tripartita.* N.O. *Compositæ.*

Synonym : Water Agrimony.

Habitat : Ditches, by waterways, and in wet places generally ; also cultivated in gardens.

Features : Erect, smooth, angular, brown-spotted stem, two to three feet high. Leaves opposite, stalked, smooth, serrate, usually in three or five segments. Flowers (July to September) in terminal heads, small, tawny. Numerous seeds, four-cornered, reflexed prickles. Root tapering, many-fibred.

Part used : Whole plant.

Action : Astringent, diuretic, diaphoretic.

Dropsy, gout and bleeding of the urinary and respiratory organs, as well as uterine hemorrhage. 1 ounce to 1 pint infusion, in wineglass doses, three or four times daily. Ginger is usually added to this herb. Hool recommends 2 ounces Burr Marigold to 1 of crushed Ginger in 3 pints of water simmered down to 1 quart, given in the above quantity five times daily, or oftener if necessary.

BUTTER-BUR. *Tussilago petasites.* N.O. *Compositæ.*

Synonym : Common Butterbur.

Habitat : Low-lying meadows and damp waysides.

Features : Stem thick, nearly one foot high. Leaves, appearing after the flowers, very large, cordate, downy underneath. Pink flowers on short stalks bloom in early spring in thick spikes. Rhizome quarter-inch thick, furrowed longitudinally, purplish-brown, pithy.

Part used : Rhizome.

Action : Stimulant, diuretic.

Now little used except locally. Was formerly valued in feverish colds and urinary complaints.

CALUMBA. *Jateorhiza calumba.* N.O. *Menispermaceæ.*

Synonym : *Cocculus palmatus,* Colombo.

Habitat : Ceylon.

Features : Root bark thick, greyish-brown outside, transverse section yellowish, vascular bundles in radiating lines. Fracture short and mealy. Very bitter and mucilaginous in taste.

Part used : Root.

Action : Tonic, febrifuge.

As a bitter tonic without astringency, in weakness of stomach function and indigestion generally. The infusion of 1 ounce of the powdered root to 1 pint of cold water is taken in two tablespoonful doses three or four times daily.

For bowel flatulence, U.S. Dispensatory gives : ½ ounce

each powdered Calumba and Ginger, 1 drachm Senna, infused in 1 pint boiling water. Dose, wineglassful three times daily.

CARDAMOMS. *Elettaria cardamomum.* N.O. *Zingiberaceæ.*

Synonym : Mysore Cardamoms, Malabar Cardamoms.
Habitat : Cultivated chiefly in Ceylon.
Features : Fruits ovoid or oblong, longitudinally furrowed, about half-inch long. Fruits yield approximately 75 per cent seeds.
Part used : Seeds.
Action : Carminative, stomachic.

As a warm, grateful aromatic in flatulence. The seeds should be crushed, and an infusion of 2 ounces to 1 pint of water taken in wineglassful doses.

CASCARA SAGRADA. *Rhamnus purshiana.* N.O. *Rhamnaceæ.*

Synonym : Sacred Bark, Chittem Bark.
Habitat : California and British Columbia.
Features : Bark in quills about three-quarter inch wide by one-sixteenth inch thick, furrowed longitudinally, purplish-brown in colour. Inner surface longitudinally striated, transversely wrinkled. Fracture pale brown, or dark brown when older. Persistently bitter taste, leather-like odour.
Older bark is preferred, younger sometimes griping.
Part used : Bark.
Action : Tonic laxative.

In habitual constipation due to sluggishness and atony of the lower bowel, and for digestive disorders generally. Doses for chronic constipation, firstly ½ to 1 teaspoonful at bedtime, afterwards 5-10 drops before each meal, of the fluid extract.

CATNEP. *Nepeta cataria.* N.O. *Labiatæ.*

Synonym : Catmint, Catnip.

Habitat : Hedgerows.

Features : Square, grey, hairy stem, up to two feet high. Leaves stalked, cordate-ovate, serrate, whitish down beneath. Flowers white, crimson dots, two-lipped, in short, dense spikes. Characteristic mint-like scent.

Part used : Herbs, leaves.

Action : Carminative, tonic, diaphoretic, anti-spasmodic.

Especially used for flatulence and digestive pains in children, and for production of perspiration in both children and adults. For diaphoretic purposes in adults, 2-tablespoonful doses of the 1 ounce to 1 pint infusion thrice daily, with a cupful at bedtime ; proportionate doses in children's complaints.

American physio-medical practice recommends blood-warm bowel injections of the infusion for babies with intestinal flatulence.

CAYENNE. *Capsicum minimum.* N.O. *Solanaceæ.*

Synonym : African Pepper, Bird Pepper, Guinea Pepper and Chillies.

Habitat : There are many varieties of the shrub, which is indigenous to India, Africa and South America.

Features : The oblong-conical shaped pods are fiery to the taste, and the numerous seeds contain a large amount of oil, which has a similar effect on the palate. The fruit itself, however, differs widely in size, colour and strength. The yellowish-red product of Sierra Leone is the most pungent, the long, bright red type from Japan being much milder.

(*Capsicum annum* is cultivated in Hungary, and fed to canaries in order to improve the appearance of the plumage. Known as "tasteless Cayenne," this is quite free from pungency.)

Part used : Dried, ripe fruit. Used for medicinal and culinary purposes.

Action : Cayenne is acknowledged as the finest stimulant in the herbal materia medica, and is, in addition, carminative, tonic, diaphoretic and rubefacient.

As a pure stimulant, the administration of Cayenne produces a natural warmth and uniform circulation, and in dyspepsia and flatulence the carminative effect is especially noticeable. As a diaphoretic it may be used whenever it is desired to open the pores and bring about increased perspiration.

Capsicum is a constituent of many of the herbal compounds, including the well-known composition powders, Thomson's formula for which will be found in the appropriate section of this book. The dose of the powdered fruit is 5-20 grains.

Coffin is a champion of the virtues of Capsicum, one of his reasons being that, unlike most of the stimulants of allopathy, it is not a narcotic.

CELANDINE. *Chelidonium majus*. N.O. *Papaveraceæ*.

Synonym : Garden Celandine, Greater Celandine.

Habitat : Uncultivated places, and close to old walls.

Features : This straggling, well-branched plant, which belongs to the poppy family, is not related either medicinally or botanically to Pilewort, which latter is commonly known as the Small or Lesser Celandine. This apparent confusion probably arose from some imagined superficial resemblance. The hairy stem of our present subject reaches a height of two feet, and exudes a saffron-yellow juice when fresh. The pinnate leaves are also slightly hairy, green above and greyish underneath, and are six to twelve inches long by two to three inches wide. The root tapers, and the yellow flowers appear in May and June singly at the end of three or four smaller stalks given off from the end of a main flower stalk. The taste is bitter and caustic, the smell disagreeable.

Part used : Herb.

Action : Alterative, diuretic and cathartic.

The infusion of 1 ounce to 1 pint of boiling water is taken in wineglassful doses three times daily, as part of the treatment for jaundice, eczema, and scrofulous diseases. The infusion is also helpful when applied directly to abrasions and bruises, and the fresh juice makes a useful application for corns and warts.

Culpeper knew of the virtues of Celandine in jaundice, and refers to it thus : "The herb or roots boiled in white wine and drunk, a few Aniseeds being boiled therewith, openeth obstructions of the liver and gall, helpeth the yellow jaundice."

CELERY. *Apium graveolens.* N.O. *Umbelliferæ.*

Synonym : Smallage.

Habitat : Moist ground near the sea.

Features : Stem smooth, one to two feet high. Main flower stalk very short, smaller flower stalks springing therefrom, whitish flowers. Seeds tiny, ovate, brown, with five paler ribs. Flavour and smell like garden celery.

Part used : Seeds.

Action : Diuretic, carminative, tonic.

Widely used as a uric acid solvent and in many forms of rheumatism in combination with suitable alteratives— see formula in this volume. Also as a tonic with Damiana. The dose is 5-30 drops of the fluid extract.

CENTAURY. *Erythræa centaurium.* N.O. *Gentianaceæ.*

Synonym : Century, Feverwort.

Habitat : Dry pastures.

Features : Stem up to one foot high. Leaves opposite, lanceolate-ovate, three to five longitudinal ribs, smooth, entire at margins. Flowers (July and August) pink, twisted anthers. Whole plant bitter to the taste.

Part used : Herb.

Action : Stomachic, bitter tonic.

In dyspepsia. Also jaundice, together with Bayberry bark. Three or four wineglass doses daily of the 1 ounce to 1 pint infusion.

R. L. Hool recommends equal parts of Centaury and Raspberry leaves in a similar infusion and dosage to above as a tonic for delicate and elderly people. He considers that Centaury "acts particularly upon the heart as a general strengthener." Coffin stresses its value in jaundice.

CHAMOMILE. *Anthemis nobilis.* N.O. *Compositæ.*

Synonym : Double Chamomile, Roman Chamomile.

Habitat : Gravelly heaths. Indigenous to Britain, and cultivated in Belgium, Germany and France.

Features : The creeping stem throws up short, leafy, flowering branches. The leaves are pinnately divided into short, hairy leaflets. Yellow centred, with a fringe of white petals, the flowers grow singly on leafless flower stalks ; the familiar double flowers are produced under cultivation. The taste is very bitter, and, in view of the resemblance which the strong, aromatic smell has to that of the apple, it is interesting to note that the name "Chamomile" is derived from the Greek, meaning "ground apple."

Part used : Flowers and herb, but the flowers are the more commonly used part.

Action : Stomachic, anti-spasmodic and tonic.

The famous "chamomile tea" is taken for nervous and bilious headache, as an aid to digestion, and for hysterical tendencies in women. The dose is up to 4 tablespoonfuls of the infusion of 1 ounce to 1 pint of water. Externally, the flower-heads make a first-rate poultice and fomentation for bruises and deep-seated inflammation, and are also used as a lotion for toothache, earache and neuralgia. In the pulverized form they may be made up with Soapwort into a shampoo, especially for fair hair.

CHICKWEED. *Stellaria media.* N.O. *Caryophyllaceæ.*

Synonym : Starweed, Star Chickweed.

Habitat : Waste places, roadsides.

Features : Stem weak, straggling, freely branched ; line of white hairs along one side only, changing direction at each pair of leaves. Leaves small, ovate, sessile above, flat stalks lower. Flowers white, very small, petals deeply cleft, singly on axils of upper leaves. Taste slightly salty.

Part used : Herb.

Action : Demulcent, emollient, pectoral.

Inflammation of the respiratory organs and internal membranes generally. One ounce of herb in 1½ pints of water simmered down to 1 pint. Dose, wineglassful every two or three hours. Used externally as a poultice for inflamed surfaces, boils, burns and skin eruptions.

CHICORY. *Cichorium intybus.* N.O. *Compositæ.*

Synonym : Succory.

Habitat : Waysides, field borders, waste land.

Features : Stem grows to three feet, upstanding, rigid, tough, many branches at obtuse angles. Lower leaves large, margins coarsely notched, projecting lobes ; upper, small, sessile, less divided. Flowers, delicate greyish-blue, many strap-like petals, stalkless, two or three together between leaves and stem. Root brownish ; reticulated white layers surround radiate, woody column.

Part used : Root.

Action : Hepatic, laxative, diuretic.

Jaundice and other liver disorders, gout and rheumatism. This root, when roasted and ground, is mixed with coffee, to the benefit of drinkers of that beverage.

CHIRETTA. *Swertia chirata.* N.O. *Gentianaceæ.*

Synonym : Brown Chirata, Chirayta, Griseb.

Habitat : Northern India.

Features : Stem purplish-brown, cylindrical below, becoming quadrangular higher up, pithy, nearly quarter-inch thick. Leaves opposite, three to seven longitudinal ribs, entire. Fruit (capsule) one-celled, two valved. Extremely bitter taste.

Part used : Whole plant.

Action : Bitter tonic.

In all cases where a tonic is indicated. With suitable hepatics and laxatives, sometimes forms part of prescriptions for liver complaints, dyspepsia and constipation.

Dose, two to four tablespoonfuls of ½ ounce to 1 pint infusion.

CINQUEFOIL. *Potentilla reptans.* N.O. *Rosaceæ.*

Synonym : Five-leaf-grass, Fivefinger.

Habitat : Meadows, pastures, waysides.

Features : Stem long and creeping, rooting at joints, as the strawberry. Leaf stalks one to two inches long with five obovate leaflets, serrate, scattered hairs, veins prominent below. Flowers (June-September) bright yellow, five petals, solitary, on long stalks from stem as the leaves.

Part used : Herb.

Action : Astringent.

Infusion of 1 ounce to 1 pint of water in wineglass doses for diarrhœa. Also as a gargle for relaxed throat. Externally, as an astringent skin lotion.

CLIVERS. *Galium aparine.* N.O. *Rubiaceæ.*

Synonym : Cleavers, Goosegrass, Catchweed, Goosebill, Hayriffe.

Habitat : Among hedges and bushes.

Features : Quadrangular stem, rough, weak but very lengthy, creeping up the hedges by little prickly hooks. Many side branches, always in pairs. Leaves small, lanceolate, in rings of six to nine round stem, with backward, bristly hairs at margins. Flowers white, very small, petals arranged like Maltese Cross ; few together on stalk rising from leaf ring. Fruit nearly globular, one-eighth inch diameter, also covered with hooked bristles. Saline taste.

Part used : Herb.

Action : Diuretic, tonic, alterative.

Obstructions of urinary organs. Hot or cold infusion of 1 ounce to 1 pint in wineglass doses frequently. Clivers is similar in action to Gravelroot, the former causing a more copious watery flow, the latter a larger proportion of solid matter. The two herbs are frequently used together.

CLOVES. *Eugenia caryophyllata.* N.O. *Myrtaceæ.*

Synonym : Clavos.

Habitat : Indigenous to the Molucca Island, cultivated in Zanzibar, Madagascar, Java, Penang.

Features : Flower buds brown ; nail-shaped, calyx tube encloses ovary containing tiny ovules ; four calyx teeth surrounded by unopened corolla consisting of four petals.

Part used : Flower buds.

Action : Stimulant, aromatic, carminative.

Combined with more specific remedies in flatulence and other affections of the alimentary tract. Is an excellent carminative to reduce griping action of purgatives. Dose, 1 to 2 tablespoonfuls of the infusion.

Coffin holds that Cloves are the most powerful of all the carminatives.

COHOSH, BLACK. *Cimicifuga racemosa.* N.O. *Ranunculaceæ.*

Synonym : Known also as Black Snakeroot.

Habitat : The dried rhizome and roots are imported from the U.S.A., to which country and Canada the plant is indigenous.

Features : Thick, hard and knotty, the root is bitter and acrid in taste, and gives off a rather nauseating smell.

Part used : Rhizome and roots.

Action : Astringent, diuretic, emmenagogue and alterative.

The decoction of 1 ounce to 1 pint (reduced from 1½ pints) of water, is administered in wineglassful doses. Its chief importance lies in the treatment of rheumatism, and the root figures frequently in herbal prescriptions for this complaint. In small doses it is useful in children's diarrhœa, and is reputed to be a remedy for St. Vitus' Dance (chorea), although its efficacy here is dubious.

Cimicifuga should be taken with care, as overdoses produce nausea and vomiting.

COLTSFOOT. *Tussilago farfara.* N.O. *Compositæ.*

Synonym : Also recognised as Coughwort and Horsehoof, the name Coltsfoot is from the shape of the leaf, which is supposed to resemble a colt's foot.

Habitat : It prefers moist, clayey soil, and is usually found growing near streams and ditches.

Features : Springing erect from the ground to a height of about eight inches, the stem is entirely covered with small brown scales and a loose cottony down. The angular, long-stalked, toothed leaves are about four inches, green above with long white hairs underneath. Large, daisy type, bright yellow flowers appear, one to each stalk, from February to April, long before the leaf growth. The taste is mucilaginous and rather astringent, the odour scarcely noticeable.

Part used : Leaves.

Action : Expectorant and demulcent.

Coltsfoot leaves are used in a decotion of 1 ounce to 1½

pints of water, simmered down to 1 pint, which is taken in teacupful doses. Its expectorant and demulcent action is of great help in cough remedies when in conjunction with pectorals such as Horehound. The leaves also form a useful constituent of asthma and whooping-cough medicines, and are smoked as a relief against asthma, bronchitis and catarrh.

These same uses were known centuries ago, as witness Culpeper : "The dry leaves are best for those that have thin rheums, and distillations upon the lungs, causing a cough, for which also the dried leaves taken as tobacco, or the root, is very good."

COMFREY. *Symphytum officinale.* N.O. *Boraginaceæ.*

Synonym : Knitbone, Nipbone.

Habitat : Damp fields and waste places ; ditch and river sides.

Features : The hairy stem is two to three feet high, freely branched, rough and angular. Egg-shaped to lance-shaped leaves, with wavy edges, hug the stem above, the lower ones having long stalks ; they are all large and hairy. The plant produces yellowish, bluish, or purplish-white flowers in May and June, all on the same side of the stem. The root is brownish-black, deeply wrinkled, greyish and horny internally. The taste is mucilaginous and sweetish, and the dried herb has an odour resembling that of tea.

Part used : Root and leaves.

Action : The roots, and to some extent the leaves, are demulcent and astringent.

The action of Comfrey is similar to that of Marsh Mallow, and consequently it is a popular cough remedy. It is also used as a fomentation in strained and inflammatory conditions of the muscles, and will promote suppuration of boils and other skin eruptions. A decoction is made by boiling ½ to 1 ounce of the crushed root in 1 quart of water, reducing to 1½ pints, and is taken in wineglass doses.

Coffin tells us the root of the plant is also "a good tonic

medicine, and acts friendly on the stomach ; very useful in cases where, from maltreatment, the mouth, the throat and stomach have become sore."

COWSLIP. *Primula veris.* N.O. *Primulaceæ.*

Synonym : Herb Peter, Paigles, Palsywort.
Habitat : Moist pastures and open places.
Features : Round, downy stem rising well above the leaves, which lie, rosette-like, on the ground. Leaves grow from the root, stalkless, undivided, velvety appearance similar to primrose leaves, but shorter and rounder. Yellow, tubular flowers bunch together on one stalk, each flower emerging from the same point, outer blossoms drooping.
Part used : Corolla.
Action : Antispasmodic, sedative.

In the reduction of involuntary spasmodic movements, restlessness and similar symptoms. Used also in insomnia. The usual herbal infusion is taken in tablespoonfuls as required.

Both cowslip and primrose were at one time prescribed for rheumatism, gout and paralysis, but their value in these diseases has long since been disproved.

CRAMP BARK. *Viburnum opulus.* N.O. *Caprifoliaceæ.*

Synonym : Guelder Rose, High Cranberry, Snowball Tree.
Habitat : Cultivated in shrubberies, etc., for decorative purposes.
Features : Very thin bark, greyish-brown outside with corky growths (lenticels), slight longitudinal crackings, laminate, light brown internally. Fracture forms flat splinters.
Part used : Bark.
Action : Antispasmodic, nervine.

As the name indicates, in cramp and other involuntary spasmodic muscular contractions. The decoction of 1 ounce to 1 pint of water (simmered from 1½ pints) is administered in 1-2 tablespoon doses.

CRANESBILL. *Geranium pratense.* N.O. *Geraniaceæ.*

Synonym :   Meadow Cranesbill.
Habitat :   Moist pasture land.
Features :   Stem up to three feet high, swollen at the joints, freely branched. Dark green leaves, almost circular in form, with five to seven much-divided leaflets, coarsely notched at edges. Seed-pod is distinctive—long, sharp-pointed, pendulous—and might be said by the imaginative to resemble a "crane's bill."
Part used :   Herb.
Action :   Astringent, tonic, diuretic.

Arrests internal and external bleeding, and exerts tonic and astringent effect on the kidneys. Decoction of equal quantities of Cranesbill and Bistort makes a good twice-daily injection against leucorrhœa. An infusion of 1 ounce Cranesbill herb to 1 pint of water may be given frequently in wineglass doses. Proportionate doses give good results in infantile diarrhœa.

> *Geranium maculatum,* or American Cranesbill, possesses similar properties to the above. The root of the former is used to some extent medicinally.

CUDWEED. *Gnaphalium uliginosum.* N.O. *Compositæ.*

Synonym :   Cotton Weed, Marsh Cudweed.
Habitat :   Wet, sandy places, particularly in East England.
Features :   Stem usually under five inches, much branched, with cottony down. Leaves smooth above, oppressed hairs underneath, about an inch long by one-fifth of an inch wide. Flowerheads small, yellowish-brown scales, in corymb form.
Part used :   Herb.
Action :   Astringent.

Of great value as a gargle for inflammation of the salivary glands of the mouth and throat generally. The 1 ounce to 1 pint infusion, in addition to being used for gargling should be taken internally in wineglassful doses.

DAMIANA. *Turnera aphrodisiaca.* N.O. *Turneraceæ.*

Habitat :   Central America.
Features :   Leaves alternate, wedge-shaped, hairy, shortly stalked, serrate, revolute. Aromatic, rather fig-like taste.
Part used : Leaves.
Action :   Aphrodisiac, tonic.

Used for its aphrodisiac qualities and general tonic effect on the nervous system. The 1 ounce to 1 pint infusion may be taken in wineglass doses thrice daily.

DANDELION. *Taraxacum officinale.* N.O. *Compositæ.*

The name of this almost ubiquitous plant is a corruption of the French "dents de lion" (lion's teeth), and refers to the coarse teeth edging the leaf.

Features :   The stem is slender, hollow, and contains the familiar milk-like juice. The long thin leaves, which are broader towards the top than at the base, are tooth-edged in a slightly backward direction. Each of the petals, of which only the central portion of the yellow, daisy-like flower is wholly composed, are strap-like in form. The roots are long, dark brown, and bitter to the taste, although not unpleasantly so.
Part used : Roots and leaves.
Action :   Diuretic, tonic, and slightly aperient.

While a Dandelion decoction of 1 ounce to 1 pint (reduced from 1½ pints) may be taken alone and drunk freely with benefit, the properties of the herb are better utilised in combination with other agents. The root is a constituent of many prescriptions for dropsical and urinary complaints, and in atonic dyspepsia and rheumatism. Contrary to widely-held belief, Dandelion root would seem to have little or no action on the liver.

The most popular use for Dandelion root, after roasting and grinding, is as a substitute for coffee, to which beverage it bears a remarkable resemblance. Prepared like coffee, but using only about half the quantity, and drunk regularly, it acts as a mild laxative in habitual constipation, without any of the disadvantages which attend coffee drinking. The fresh leaf is best taken in salads. Juice of either flower stalk or leaf, freshly gathered, is of help in removing warts.

DEVIL'S BIT. *Scabiosa succisa*. N.O. *Compositæ*.

Synonym : Ofbit.
Habitat : Heaths and pastures.
Features : Stem up to eighteen inches, slender, hairy, well-branched. Leaves opposite, oval-lanceolate, slightly serrate, nearly sessile ; root leaves stalked, ovoid, smooth at margins. Flowers dark purple, on long stalk, florets bunched together.

The common name is derived from the root, which appears to have been bitten off at the end, with which vandalism "the devil" is credited.
Part used : Herb.
Action : Demulcent, diaphoretic.

Included in formulæ for coughs and feverish conditions generally. A 1 ounce to 1 pint infusion may be taken warm in wineglassful doses frequently.

DILL. *Peucedanum graveolens*. N.O. *Compositæ*.

Synonym : Dill Fruit, Dill Seed, Eneldo.
Habitat : Waste places ; also seen growing wild in gardens.
Features : Stem erect, smooth, channelled, covered with exuded glaucous matter. Leaves alternate, twice pinnate. Flowers in June, terminal umbels. Fruits very small, compressed oval, marked on back in three ridges, with three dark lines (oil cells) between. Taste is distinctive, but recalls caraway.

The Indian Dill differs from our European variety in the essential oil contained in the seeds.
Part used : Dried ripe fruits.
Action : Carminative, stomachic, diaphoretic.

The well-known and widely used Dillwater is a sound remedy for children's digestive disorders, particularly wind in stomach or bowels. Dose, 1 to 8 drachms. The oil is also given in 1 to 5 drop doses.

ELDER. *Sambucus nigra.* N.O. *Caprifoliaceæ.*

Synonym : Black Elder, European Elder.

Habitat : Woods and hedges throughout Europe.

Features : This familiar small tree, twelve to twenty feet high, has young branches containing light, spongy pith, with a bark that is light grey and corky externally. The leaves are opposite, deep green and smooth. Creamy-white, flat-topped masses of flowers bloom in July, to be followed by the decorative, drooping bunches of purplish-black, juicy berries. Country folk aptly limit our English summer when they say that it does not arrive until the Elder is in full blossom, and ends when the berries are ripe !

Part used : Flowers.

Action : Diaphoretic, emollient, alterative, diuretic.

These properties of the flowers are obtained from infusions of 1 ounce to 1 pint of water in wineglass doses. It is used, often in conjunction with Peppermint and Yarrow, chiefly for the reduction of feverish colds, but inflamed conditions of the eyes are also found to yield to bathing with the warm Elder flower infusion. Although the medicinal qualities are weaker in the berries than in the flowers, the popular Elder berry wine is widely used as part of the treatment for colds and influenza.

An ointment made from the leaves has been of help to sufferers from chilblains.

ELECAMPANE. *Inula helenium.* N.O. *Compositæ.*

Synonym : Aunée, Scabwort.

Habitat : Moist meadows and pasture land.

Features : The stem, growing up to three feet, is branched, furrowed, and downy above ; egg-shaped, serrate leaves embrace the stem. The calyx is also egg-shaped and leafy, and the flowers, blooming in July and August, are large, solitary and terminal, brilliantly yellow in colour. The root is light grey, hard, horny and cylindrical. The whole plant is similar in appearance to the horseradish its taste is bitter and acrid, and the odour reminiscent of camphor.

Part used : Root.

Action : Diaphoretic, expectorant and diuretic.

In combination with other remedies it is made up into cough medicines, and can be of service in pulmonary disorders generally. Skilfully compounded, slight alterative and tonic qualities are noticed. Wineglass doses are taken of a 1 ounce to 1 pint (reduced) decoction.

These modest present-day claims for Elecampane are far exceeded by Culpeper's exuberance. In his view, the root "warms a cold and windy stomach or the pricking therein, and stitches in the side caused by the spleen ; helps the cough, shortness of the breath, and wheezing of the lungs. . . . Profitable for those that have their urine stopped. . . . Resisteth poison, and stayeth the venom of serpents, as also of putrid and pestilential fevers, and the plague itself." When we are also told by the same author that it kills and expels worms, fastens loose teeth, arrests dental decay, cleanses the skin from morphew, spots and blemishes, we realize in what esteem Elecampane was held in the seventeenth century ! But here again germs of truth are hidden among manifold exaggerations.

ERYNGO. *Eryngium maritimum.* N.O. *Umbelliferæ.*

Synonym : Commonly known as Sea Holly and Sea Eryngo.

Habitat : The plant is seen only on the sand dunes of the sea shore.

Features : A pale greenish-blue bloom is characteristic of the erect, smooth stem, which grows to nearly one foot. Stiff, wavy, roundish leaves are roughly divided into three short, broad lobes, with beautiful veins and sharp teeth at the margins. Root leaves have stalks, but those from the stem are sessile. Blooming from July to September, the bright, pale blue flowers form a dense, round head at the end of branches. The blackish-brown roots, long, thin and cylindrical, are topped with the bristly remnants of the leaf stalks, and have a sweetish, mucilaginous taste.

Part used : The root is the only part of the plant recognised in herbalism.

Action : Eryngo root is a diaphoretic, diuretic and expectorant.

It is mostly prescribed for bladder disorders, such as difficult and painful micturivion, and also forms part of the treatment for uterine irritation.

Richard Lawrence Hool, of the British and American Physio-Medical Association, advises it in "sluggishness of the liver with uric acid accumulations," prepared as follows :

> "Sea Holly . 1 ounce
> Wild Carrot . 1 ounce.

"Boil in 1½ pints of water down to 1 pint ; strain, and take a wineglassful four times a day. In cases of jaundice take :

> "Sea Holly . 1 ounce
> Barberry bark . ½ ounce

"Boil in 1 quart of new milk for 10 minutes. Strain, and take two wineglassfuls every three hours." He adds : "Most obstinate cases have been known to yield to this remedy in from 7 to 14 days."

EYEBRIGHT. *Euphrasia officinalis.* N.O. *Scrophulariaceæ.*

Synonym : Birdeye, Brighteye.

Habitat : Plentiful on commons, heaths, and in meadows, as well as on sea cliffs, but varies considerably in growth and development with the richness of the soil.

Features : The stems are four to six inches long, and under suitable soil conditions, branched below. The lower leaves are opposite each other, and alternate higher up the stem, small, dark green, lanceolate or nearly rhomboid above, deeply cut, proceeding directly from the stem. The flowers are small, axillary, and range in hue between white and purple, while some are delicately variegated with yellow. The taste is bitter, salty and slightly astringent.

Action : Astringent and tonic.

This herb, as its name indicates, is valued mainly as an application in inflammation and weakness of the eyes, and is frequently combined with Golden Seal to make an excellent lotion for this purpose. A large pinch of the herb should be infused with sufficient boiling water for each application. The eyebath should be freshly filled for each eye, care being taken to strain thoroughly before using the tepid lotion.

Euphrasia is also employed externally to arrest hemorrhages.

FENNEL. *Fœniculum dulce.* N.O. *Umbelliferæ.*

Synonym : Hinojo.

Habitat : Chalk cliffs and downs.

Features : Stem erect, three to four feet, striated, smooth, freely branched. Leaves thrice pinnate, awl-shaped leaflets. Flowers (July and August) golden yellow, in broad, terminal umbels. Fruit oblong, cylindrical, slightly curved, half-inch long by one-tenth inch broad. Taste and smell, sweetish and aromatic.

Part used : Seeds.

Action : Carminative, stomachic, stimulant, diaphoretic.

In prescriptions where the above-mentioned properties are needed in mild form. These seeds appear in the formula for the well-known Compound Liquorice Powder. May be taken in the usual infusion.

FEVERFEW. *Chrysanthemum parthenium.* N.O. *Compositæ.*

Synonym : Featherfew, Featherfoil, *Pyrethrum parthenium.*
Habitat : Waste places, hedges.
Features : Stem one and a half feet high, erect, finely furrowed, hairy, branches towards top. Leaves alternate, bipinnatifid, serrate edges, very short hairs, about four and a half by two and a half inches ; leaf stalk flat above, convex below. Numerous flowers (June and July), yellow disc, white petals, each on stalk. Taste, very unpleasant.
Part used : Herb.
Action : Aperient, carminative.

Assists in promotion of the menses and in the expulsion of worms. Also given in hysterical conditions. Infusion of 1 ounce to 1 pint boiling water, wineglassful doses.

FRINGE-TREE. *Chionanthus virginica.* N.O. *Oleaceæ.*

Synonym : Old Man's Beard, Snowdrop Tree.
Habitat : U.S.A.
Features : A small tree with snow-white flowers which hang down like fringe—hence the common name and synonyms. Root about one-eighth inch thick, dull brown with irregular concave scars on outer surface, inside smooth, yellowish-brown. Fracture short, inner layer shows projecting bundles of stone cells. Very bitter taste.
Part used : Root bark.
Action : Alterative, hepatic, diuretic, tonic.

In stomach and liver disorders, and poor digestive functioning generally. Also finds a place in gall-stone prescriptions and those for certain female disorders, in which latter Pulsatilla is another frequent constituent. The 1 ounce to 1 pint infusion is taken internally in 1-4 tablespoonful doses, and is applied as lotion and injection.

FUMITORY. *Fumaria officinalis.* N.O. *Fumariaceæ.*

Synonym : Earth Smoke.

Habitat : Roadsides, fields, gardens.

Features : Stem weak, brittle, sometimes erect, sometimes trailing, six to twelve inches long. Leaves alternate, twice pinnate, bluish-green. Flowers (May to November) reddish-rose, several on stalk.

Part used : Herb.

Action : Slightly tonic, duretic, aperient.

For stomach and liver disorders and minor skin blemishes. Infusion of 1 ounce to 1 pint may be taken freely.

GENTIAN. *Gentiana lutea.* N.O. *Gentianaceæ.*

Habitat : Grows abundantly throughout France, Spain, and large areas of Central Europe.

Part used : Large quantities of *Gentiana lutea* root are imported into this country as it is preferred to the English variety (*Gentiana campestris*—see below) for no very apparent therapeutic reason. It is certain, however, that Gentian root, of whichever kind, is the most popular of all herbal tonics and stomachics—and deservedly so.

Features : *Gentiana lutea* root is cylindrical in form, half to one inch thick, and ringed in the upper portion, the lower being longitudinally wrinkled. It is flexible and tough, internally spongy and nearly white when fresh, an orange-brown tint and strong distinctive odour developing during drying. The taste is extremely bitter.

A decoction of 1 ounce to 1 pint (reduced from 1½ pints) of water, given in wineglass doses, will be found very helpful in dyspepsia and loss of tone, or general debility of the digestive organs. One of the effects of the medicine is to stimulate the nerve-endings of taste, thus increasing the flow of gastric juice. As a simple bitter it may be given in all cases when a tonic is needed.

The English Gentian (also known locally as Baldmoney and Felwort) grows to six inches high and is branched above. Leaves opposite, ovate-lanceolate above and ovate-spatulate below, entire margins. Flowers are bluish-purple. The whole herb may be used for the same purposes as the foreign root, although here also the root contains the more active principles.

GINGER, WILD. *Asarum canadense.* N.O. *Aristolochiaceæ.*

Synonym : Canadian Snake Root.

Habitat : Woods and shady places in North America.

Features : Imported rhizome, slender, about four inches long by one-eighth inch thick, quadrangular, greyish to purplish brown, wrinkled ; fracture short ; rootlets whitish. Pungent, bitter taste.

Part used : Rhizome.

Action : Stimulant, carminative, expectorant, diaphoretic.

As a carminative in digestive and intestinal pains, and as a stimulant in colds and amenorrhœa resulting therefrom. An infusion of ½ ounce of the powdered rhizome to 1 pint boiling water is taken hot for stimulative purposes, and blood warm as a carminative. Dose of the dry powder, 20 to 30 grains.

Practitioners of the American Physio-Medical School hold that this root exerts a direct influence upon the uterus, and prescribe it as a parturient when nervous fatigue is observed.

GOLDEN SEAL. *Hydrastis canadensis.* N.O. *Ranunculaceæ.*

Synonym : Orange Root, Yellow Root.

Habitat :   This valuable plant appears, according to Coffin, to have been first discovered and used by the aborigines of North America. It is indigenous to that part of the world.

Features :   Golden Seal is found growing to a height of one to two feet in rich, moist and shady soils. The leaves are alternate, the lower one stalked, the upper one sessile. Both are unequally toothed, and have from three to seven acute lobes. White and red single terminal flowers bloom in April. The root is short, knotty with the bases of stems, and covered with many rootlets. The taste is very bitter, and the scent strong and unpleasant.

Part used : Golden Seal was so named by the followers of Thomson, who first used the root about 1845, since when it has figured prominently in herbal practice.

Action :   Tonic, alterative, and laxative.

Golden Seal has proved itself to be a very valuable remedy in digestive disorders and in debilitated conditions of mucous membranes. Its use is indicated in various gastric complaints, and it may be taken with advantage by most dyspeptics in doses of 10 grains of the powdered root.

Hydrastis is also given in conjunction with Lime flowers and Valerian to reduce blood pressure.

GRAVEL ROOT. *Eupatorium purpureum.* N.O. *Compositæ.*

Synonym : *Eupatorium purpureum* is also called Gravel Weed and Queen of the Meadow, from which the medicinal "Gravel Root" is obtained.

Habitat :   Gravel Root is a native of the United States, and must not be confused with the English Queen of the Meadow or Meadowsweet (*Spiræa ulmaria*).

Features : Our present subject is a member of the Boneset (*Eupatorium perfoliatum*) family, and sometimes reaches six feet in height at full growth. It is peculiar for a purple band about an inch broad round the leaf joint. Pale purple to white flowers bloom in August and September. The rhizome, as the medicinal "root" should more properly be termed, is hard and tough,

35

up to an inch thick, with a nearly white wood and thin grey-brown bark. Short, lateral branches give off thin, tough root several inches long.

Part used : Root.

Action :   Diuretic and stimulant.

Gravel root is much prescribed for cases of stone in the bladder and certain other troubles of the kidneys and urinary apparatus. A decoction of 1 ounce of the root to 1 pint (reduced from 1½ pints) of water is made, and taken in wineglass doses. Gravel root is also met with in nervine formulæ, in which its tonic properties are recognised.

The American physio-medical or "Thomsonite" M.D., F. H. England, has said that Gravel Root "induces very little stimulation. It expends nearly all its influence on the kidneys, bladder and uterus. It probably influences the whole sympathetic nervous system. Its use promotes the flow of urine as scarcely anything else will."

GRINDELIA. *Grindelia camporum.* N.O. *Compositæ.*

Synonym : *G. robusta, G. squarrosa,* Gum Plant, Hardy or Scaly Grindelia.

Habitat :   Indigenous to western regions of North America, and imported from California.

Features :   Leaves broad, narrowing at base, brittle, smooth, serrate, approximately three inches long by half an inch to one inch broad. Flower heads globular, florets yellow, scales of involucre reflexed. Bitterish taste.

Part used : Herb.

Action :   Anti-asthmatic, tonic, diuretic.

Widely prescribed for asthma and bronchitis, and often combined with Euphorbia and Yerba Santa for the former complaint. The paroxysms are quickly reduced both in sharpness and frequency. Figures prominently in the American herbal materia medica.

GROUND IVY. *Glechoma hederacea.* N.O. *Labiatæ.*

Synonym : Alehoof, Gill-go-Over-the-Ground, Haymaids, Run-away Jack.

Habitat : Woods and shady places, near old walls and under hedges.

Features : This ivy, as its common name and second synonym convey, creeps along the ground. The quadrangular, unbranched stem is six inches or so long. Two kidney-shaped leaves appear opposite each other at every joint. They are deeply crenate, the upper leaves purplish in colour and paler underneath. The roots issue at the corners of the jointed stalks, and the two-lipped, purplish flowers bloom three or four together in the axils of the upper leaves. The taste is bitter and acrid, the odour strong and aromatic.

Part used : The whole herb.

Action : Astringent, tonic, diuretic.

It is applicable to kidney disorders and dyspepsia. It was formerly valued as an antiscorbutic, but with advances in food distribution, this property is now rarely considered. In conjunction with Yarrow or Chamomile flowers an excellent poultice may be made for application to abscesses and gatherings. The infusion of 1 ounce of the herb to 1 pint of boiling water is taken in wineglass doses.

GROUNDSEL. *Senecio vulgaris.* N.O. *Compositæ.*

Common name originates from the Anglo-Saxon, meaning "ground glutton," a reference to the speed at which the plant spreads.

Habitat : A garden weed.

Features : Erect, angular, branched stem as high as nine inches. Leaves sessile, oblong ; short, toothed lobes. Flowers small, yellow, with slender, black-tipped involucral scales ; florets tubular. Salty taste.

Part used : Herb.

Action : Diuretic, hepatic.

Relief of biliary pains in 2 ounce doses of the 1 ounce to 1 pint infusion. A stronger infusion acts as a purgative and emetic.

HEARTSEASE. *Viola tricolor.* N.O. *Violaceæ.*

Synonym : Wild Pansy.

Habitat : Cultivated fields.

Features : Stem short, square, smooth, branched. Leaves ovate-lanceolate, crenate. Flowers in June, petals of differing sizes, usually wholly yellow but occasionally purple upper petals with dark stripes on lower ; single, violet-like flower to each flower stalk. Three carpel fruit.

Part used : Herb.

Action : Diaphoretic, diuretic.

The mildness of action makes it applicable in infantile skin eruptions, for which the ounce to pint infusion is given in doses according to age.

It has been said that the medicine will ward off asthmatic and epileptic convulsions, but there would appear to be no reliable confirmation of this. The claim may have originated with Culpeper, who writes, concerning Heartsease : "The spirit of it is excellently good for the convulsions in children, as also for falling sickness, and a gallant remedy for the inflammations of the lungs and breast, pleurisy, scabs, itch, etc."

HOLY THISTLE. *Carbenia benedicta.* N.O. *Compositæ.*

Synonym : Carduus benedictus, Blessed Thistle.

Features : Thomas Johnson, in his edition of Gerard's Herbal, published in 1636, gives us the following description of this member of the familiar thistle family : "The stalks of Carduus benedictus are round, rough and pliable, and being parted into diverse branches, do lie flat on the ground ; the leaves are jagged round about and full of harmless prickles in the edges ; the heads on the top of the stalks are set with and environed with sharp prickling leaves, out of which standeth a yellow flower ; the seed is long and set with hairs at the top like a beard ; the root is white and parted into strings ; the whole herb, leaves and stalks, and also the heads, are covered with a thin down."

Action :   Although more popular among the old herbalists than among those of to-day, Holy Thistle is still valued for its tonic, stimulant and diaphoretic properties.

Mainly used in digestive troubles, the 1 ounce to 1 pint infusion, given warm in wineglass doses several times daily, is also found capable of breaking up obstinate colds. As it is held to stimulate the mammary glands, the infusion has been given with the object of promoting the secretion of milk.

Tilke is enthusiastic in his praise of the herb : "I have found it such a clarifier of the blood, that by drinking an infusion once or twice a day, sweeted with honey, instead of tea, it would be a perfect cure for the headache, or what is commonly called the meagrims." The same writer recommends it as a salad "instead of watercresses."

The medicinal use of Holy Thistle goes back far beyond the days of Tilke, or even Johnson. William Turner, Domestic Physician to the Lord Protector Somerset in the reign of King Edward VI, in his Herbal published 1568, agrees with Tilke that the herb is "very good for the headache and the megram."

HOPS. *Humulus lupulus.* N.O. *Urticaceæ.*

Habitat :   Extensively farmed for the brewing industry, and is found growing wild in hedges and open woods.

Features :   Stem rough, very long, will twist round any adjacent support. Leaves in pairs, stalked, rough, serrate, cordate, three- or five-lobed. Flowers or catkins (more correctly called strobiles) consist of membranous scales, yellowish-green, roundish, reticulate-veined, nearly half-inch long, curving over each other. These are the fertile flowers which are used medicinally and industrially.

Action :   Tonic, diuretic.

As a tonic in prescriptions for debility, nervous dyspepsia, and general atony. Although usually given in combination with other herbs, the ounce to pint infusion of hops taken thrice daily makes quite a good tonic medicine for those feeling "run-down." Lying on a pillow stuffed with hops is an old-fashioned way of dealing with insomnia.

HOREHOUND. *Marrubium vulgare.* N.O. *Labiatæ.*

Synonym : Hoarhound.
Habitat : Horehound flourishes in dry, and particularly chalky waste ground.
Features : It grows to a height of one and a half to two feet. The bluntly four-cornered stem sends out spreading branches covered with white, woolly hair. The leaves, also spread with the soft hair, are egg-shaped and deeply toothed, the lower ones stalked, those above sessile. The small, white flowers appear during July in thick rings just above the upper leaves.
Part used : The whole plant.
Action : Aromatic and bitter, having expectorant and slight diuretic action.

Horehound is probably the best known of all herbal pectoral remedies, and is undoubtedly effective in coughs, colds and pulmonary complaints. The whole herb is infused in 1 ounce quantities to 1 pint of water, and taken frequently in wineglass doses.

The refreshing and healthy Horehound Beer or Ale is brewed from this herb, and a Horehound candy is made which, when properly prepared, is one of the best of "cough sweets."

Coffin speaks highly of the tonic and expectorant qualities of Horehound, and its latter virtue has certainly been known for nearly three hundred years, as Culpeper tells us that "it helpeth to expectorate tough phlegm from the chest."

HOREHOUND, BLACK. *Ballota nigra.* N.O. *Labiatæ.*

Synonym : Crantz, *Marrubium nigrum.*
Habitat : Hedgerows, waste ground.
Features : Stem stiff, erect, freely branched, up to four feet high. Leaves greyish-green, upper ovate, lower cordate, in pairs, each pair pointing in opposite direction to next pair, crenate, hairy, stalked. Flowers (July and August) purplish, labiate, in rings just above leaves. Disagreeable odour.
Part used : Herb.
Action : Stimulant, expectorant, diaphoretic, antispasmodic.

Coughs, colds and bronchial complaints generally. Hool prefers this herb to the white Horehound (*Marrubium vulgare*), and makes wide claims on its behalf. He recommends it in the treatment of consumption, various menstrual troubles, and parturition—in the last-named instance combined with Motherwort. "In chronic coughs, accompanied by spitting of blood," he tells us, "it will be found most excellent, either of itself or combined with other reliable remedies such as Lobelia, Marshmallow, Hyssop, etc."

HORSERADISH. *Cochlearia armoracia.* N.O. *Cruciferæ.*

Habitat : Indigenous to England and Eastern Europe.
Features : Root whitish, cylindrical, about one foot long by three-quarters of an inch through. Taste and odour pungent, irritant, mustard-like.
Part used : Root.
Action : Stimulant, diaphoretic, diuretic, emetic.

Used as a digestive. Its stimulant and diuretic properties are said to be of value in the treatment of dropsy, but it is rarely prescribed by modern herbalists.

Coffin recommends :

"Fresh Horseradish root, sliced . 1 oz.
Mustard seeds, bruised . . ½ oz.
Boiling water . . . 1 pint

41

"Let it stand in a covered vessel for four hours, then strain. Dose, three tablespoonfuls three times a day. Diuretic and stimulant. Useful in dropsies, especially those occurring after scarlet fevers and intermittents."

HYSSOP. *Hyssopus officinalis.* N.O. *Labiatæ.*

Habitat : Cultivated in gardens.

Features : Stem woody, to a height of about two feet. Leaves opposite, small, nearly sessile, lanceolate, hairy at margins. Flowers bluish-purple, in small axillary clusters on one side. Camphor-like odour.

Part used : Herb.

Action : Stimulant, pectoral, carminative, diaphoretic, febrifuge.

In cough and cold prescriptions, particularly for whooping cough, and in other troubles of infancy. The 1 ounce to 1 pint infusion is given in wineglass doses, or according to age.

ICELAND MOSS. *Cetraria islandica.* N.O. *Lichenes.*

Synonym : Cetraria, Iceland Lichen.

Habitat : Among other moss and grass in Sweden.

Features : Thallus about three inches high, branched, leafy, grey or light brown, channelled, terminates in flattened lobes, fringed with small papillæ, tiny white spots on under surface. When wet, smell resembles seaweed.

Part used : Lichen.

Action : Demulcent, nutritive, tonic.

Chronic bronchial catarrh, pulmonary complaints. Nutrient properties of considerable value. Relieves obstinate coughs. The moss should be carefully washed before preparing the decoction of 1 ounce to 1½ pints of water simmered to 1 pint. Dose, wineglassful.

JUNIPER. *Juniperus communis.* N.O. *Coniferæ.*

Habitat : This freely-branched, evergreen shrub may be seen growing on dry heaths and mountain slopes to a height of from two to five feet.

Features : The leaves open in whorls of three, are glaucous and concave above, keeled underneath. The berries are blue-black, globular, and a quarter to half-inch in diameter. An acrid taste, and a characteristic odour resembling that of turpentine, are noticeable.

Part used : Every part of the shrub is medicinal, but the dried, ripe fruit or berries only are used in modern practice.

Action : Diuretic, stimulant and carminative.

An infusion of 1 ounce of the berries to 1 pint of water may be taken freely in wineglassful doses.

As a reliable tonic diuretic, the medicine is much appreciated in kidney and bladder disorders, whether acute or chronic. Although frequently successful when taken alone, it is more usually prescribed with other agents such as Parsley Piert, Uva Ursi, and Buchu. The berries are sometimes included with suitable alteratives in formulæ for rheumatic complaints.

It is on account of the Juniper Berries used in its manufacture that gin is so frequently recommended when a diuretic is needed. However, one authority at least, Dr. Coffin, considers that "the better plan . . . is to eschew the gin, and make a tea of the berries" ! The same writer tells us that if Juniper boughs are burnt to ashes and the ashes put into water, "a medicine will be obtained that has cured the dropsy in an advanced stage."

KNAPWEED. *Centaurea nigra.* N.O. *Compositæ.*

Synonym : Hard-head, Hard-hack, Ironweed (these due to its resistance to the mower's scythe), Black Ray Thistle, Star Thistle.

Habitat : Pastures and meadows.

Features : Stem grows from one to two feet, angular, tough, very much branched on alternate sides. Leaves dull green, hard appearance, downy underneath, irregularly notched edges, upper sessile, lower stalked. Flowers thistle-shaped ; reddish-purple, hair-like petals grow from nearly black, scaly knob. Fruit without pappus, surrounded by bristles. Taste, slightly salty.

Part used : Herb.

Action :   Tonic, diaphoretic, diuretic.

As a general tonic for most of the purposes for which Gentian is used. Knapweed is held in some quarters to equal Gentian in all-round efficacy, but the latter is much more frequently prescribed. The ounce to pint infusion is taken in wineglass doses.

LADIES' MANTLE. *Alchemilla vulgaris.* N.O. *Rosaceæ.*

Synonym : Lion's Foot.

Habitat :   Hedgerows and waysides.

Features :   Whole plant covered with silky hairs. Leaves rounded, about two inches across, nine blunt, serrate lobes, on long stalks. Greenish flowers, without petals, bloom in small clusters from forked stem. Astringent, saliva-drying taste.

Part used : Herb.

Action :   Astringent, nervine, antispasmodic.

In excessive menstruation and flooding, as well as spasmodic nervous complaints. Decoction of 1 ounce to 1½ pints water simmered to 1 pint is used as an injection in the menstrual disorders. The 1 ounce to 1 pint infusion may be taken internally in teacupful doses as required.

LADIES' SLIPPER. *Cypripedium pubescens.* N.O. *Orchidaceæ.*

Synonym : American Valerian, Mocassin Flower, Nerveroot, Noah's Ark.

Habitat :   United States of America.

Features :   Flower supposed to resemble a lady's shoe in form. Rhizome about quarter-inch diameter, many cup-shaped scars on top surface ; wavy, thickly-matted roots underneath. Fracture short and white.

Part used : Rhizome.

Action : Antispasmodic, tonic, nervine.

Combined with other tonics in the relief of neuralgia, and to allay pain generally. Of use in hysteria and other nervous disorders. Dose, 1 drachm of the powdered rhizome. Like other medicines of a similar nature, it is of little use unless the cause of the nervous excitement is traced and removed.

The remarks of Rafinesque, then Professor of Medical Botany in the University of Transylvania, are interesting in view of the "orthodox" attitude towards remedies of the herbalists : "I am enabled to introduce, for the first time, this beautiful genus into our materia medica ; all the species are equally remedial. They have long been known to the Indians, who called them mocassin flower, and were used by the empyrics of New England, particularly Samuel Thomson. Their properties, however, have been tested and confirmed by Dr. Hales, of Troy ; Dr. Tully, of Albany, etc. . . . They produce beneficial effects in all nervous diseases and hysterical affections by allaying pain, quieting the nerves and promoting sleep. They are preferable to opium in many cases, having no baneful or narcotic effect."

Professor Rafinesque, however, goes even further than would Thomson and his successors when he announces that "all the species are equally remedial."

LILY-OF-THE-VALLEY. *Convallaria majalis.* N.O. *Liliaceæ.*

Synonym : Convallaria, May Lily.

Habitat : Grows wild in shady places in some of the English counties, but is rarely found in many others ; scarcely ever seen wild in Scotland and Ireland. Commonly cultivated in gardens.

Features : Leaves approximately five inches by two inches, broadly lanceolate, entire at edges, dark green, with parallel veins. Flowers small, sweet-scented, white, bell-shaped, pendulous, on distinct (eight to twelve-stalked) flower stem. Rhizome slender, cylindrical, pale brown, with eight to ten long, branched rootlets at each joint, internodes about two inches long.

Part used : Whole plant.

Action : Cardiac tonic, diuretic.

Enhances muscular functioning of heart and arteries, and is consequently used in cardiac debility. Has been recommended in dropsy. This herb is one of the substitutes for the digitalis of the allopaths, but it must be taken only in the prescribed doses, as larger quantities may result in purging and emesis. Dose, 1 tablespoonful of the $\frac{1}{2}$ ounce to 1 pint boiling water infusion.

LIME FLOWERS. *Tilia europæa.* N.O. *Liliaceæ.*

Synonym : Linden Flowers.

Habitat : The large tree is seen frequently as a decorative bordering to avenues and drives in town and country.

Features : Leaves cordate, doubly serrate, hairy underneath. Three to six yellowish-white flowers on each flower stalk ; the two anther cells are separated on short divergent stalks at the tip of the many stamens.

Part used : Flowers.

Action : Nervine, stimulant.

A popular remedy for chronic catarrhal conditions following colds, and is also given for nervous headaches and hysterical tendencies. The infusion is 1 drachm in 1 pint of boiling water, and bed-time baths in equivalent strength will sometimes help those suffering from insomnia.

LIQUORICE. *Glycyrrhiza glabra.* N.O. *Leguminosæ.*

Synonym : Licorice.

Habitat : Cultivated in gardens and fields.

Features : Stem erect, striated, with few branches. Leaves alternate, ovate, veined. Flowers (August) purple, pea-like. Root greyish-brown externally, yellowish and fibrous inside ; transverse section shows radiate structure. Taste sweetish.

Spanish and Russian roots contain large amounts of rhizome, which is decidedly less sweet than the root proper and can be recognised by a central pith. Russian and Persian varieties have a red-brown scaly exterior, and are slightly bitter and acrid.

Part used : Root.

Action : Demulcent, pectoral, emollient, expectorant.

Well-known remedy for coughs and chest complaints, frequently with linseed. A decoction of 1 ounce of the root to 1½ pints of water reduced to 1 pint, with a teaspoonful of linseed and lemon juice as desired, may be drunk freely.

LOBELIA. *Lobelia inflata.* N.O. *Campanulaceæ.*

Synonym : Indian Tobacco, Pukeweed, Emetic Weed.

Habitat : North America ; cultivated in Salt Lake City.

Features : A biennial herb, in height from twelve to eighteen inches, the stem is angular and slightly hairy. One to three inches long, the leaves are alternate, sessile, and ovate-lanceolate, with small, whitish glands on the edge. The fruit is in the form of a flat, oval capsule, which contains ovate-oblong seeds about one eighth of an inch long, brown in colour, with a reticulated, pitted surface. The root is fibrous, and the plant bears a small blue, pointed flower. The taste is burning and acrid like tobacco, the odour slight.

Part used : Herb and seeds are used.

Action : Emetic, stimulant, antispasmodic, expectorant, and diaphoretic.

Lobelia inflata has for many years been one of the most widely discussed and hotly debated articles used in medicine. While many herbalists contend that it is the most valuable of all botanic remedies, official medicine in England classifies it as a poison. Herbalists who use Lobelia insist that it is most certainly not a poison, and that it can be administered by them in large doses with perfect safety. They use it chiefly as an emetic, and, as its administration brings about the prompt removal of accumulations of mucus, the action in bronchial complaints is speedy and beneficial. Coffin's comments in this connection are enthusiastic : "Lobelia is decidedly the most certain and efficient emetic known, and is at the same time safe in its operations. Unlike most emetics from the mineral kingdom, it produces its specific effect without corroding the stomach or producing morbid irritation and inflammation of the mucous membrane of this organ, which are so common in the use of antimony, zinc, and the sulphate of copper. Lobelia may emphatically be said to 'operate in unison with the laws of life'."

In view of the controversy surrounding its use, the history of Lobelia is interesting. North American Indians had apparently long been acquainted with its properties, but its first introduction to general use was due to the efforts of the famous American, Samuel Thomson. His disciple, Dr. Coffin, brought the herb to this country and used it extensively in his practice for over forty years, apparently with great success "in almost every form of disease, and from the tender infant to the aged," to quote Coffin himself. In both America and Britain herbalists have been tried on charges of causing death by administering Lobelia, but in no instance has a verdict been obtained against them.

MANDRAKE, AMERICAN.   *Podophyllum peltatum.*
N.O. *Berberidaceæ.*

Synonym : May Apple, Racoonberry, Wild Lemon.

Habitat : A common plant in the United States and Canada, the root is imported into this country in large quantities for medicinal purposes.

Features : The rhizome (as the part used should more strictly be termed) is reddish-brown in colour, fairly smooth, and has knotty joints at distances of about two inches. The fracture shows whitish and mealy.

American Mandrake is an entirely different plant from White Bryony or English Mandrake, dealt with elsewhere. Preparations of the rhizome of the American Mandrake are found in practice to be much more effective than those of the resin. This is one of the many confirmations of one of the basic postulates of herbal medicine—the nearer we can get to natural conditions the better the results. Therapeutic principles are never the same when taken from their proper environment.

Podophyllum is a very valuable hepatic, and a thorough but slow-acting purgative. Correctly compounded with other herbs it is wonderfully effective in congested conditions of the liver, and has a salutary influence on other parts of the system, the glands in particular being helped to normal functioning. Although apparently unrecognised in Coffin's day, the modern natural healer highly appreciates the virtues of this medicine and has many uses for it.

As American Mandrake is so powerful in certain of its actions, and needs such skilful combination with other herbs, it should not be used by the public without the advice of one experienced in prescribing it to individual needs.

MARIGOLD. *Calendula officinalis.* N.O. *Compositæ.*

Synonym : Calendula, *Caltha officinalis,* Marygold.
Habitat : Common in English gardens; native of South America.
Features : Stem angular, hairy up to one foot high. Lower leaves stalked, spatulate, upper sessile, all hairy. Flowerheads yellow, the tubular florets sterile. Fruit semicircular, angular, rough, no pappus. Taste bitter, smell unpleasantly strong.
Part used : Herb, flowers.
Action : Diaphoretic, stimulant, antispasmodic.

The infusion of 1 ounce of the flowers or herb to 1 pint boiling water is prescribed both for internal use in 1-2 tablespoonful doses, and externally as a lotion for chronic ulcers and varicose veins. The infusion is also given to children (in doses according to age) suffering from measles and other feverish and eruptive complaints. Sprained muscles gain relief from the hot fomentation. Marigold is frequently combined with Witch Hazel when a lotion is required.

MARSHMALLOW. *Althæa officinalis.* N.O. *Malvaceæ.*

Synonym : Guimauve, Mallards, Schloss Tea.

Habitat : Marshes near the sea.

Features : This erect plant grows to a height of three feet, and is distinguishable from the Common Mallow by the velvety down covering the stem and leaves. Stems are round, the soft leaves being five-lobed below and three-lobed above. The pinkish-blue flowers appear in luxuriant axillar panicles between July and September. Roots are thick and fleshy, resembling those of the parsnip, and greyish-white outside, white and fibrous internally. The taste is mucilaginous and unpleasant, with only a very slight odour. The roots should be stored in a very dry place, or a yellowish matter of disagreeable smell will form.

Part used : Root and leaves.

Action : The root is preferred, as the demulcent, emollient, diuretic and expectorant properties are present here in greater strength.

Marshmallow, usually in combination with other remedies, is taken internally for coughs, colds and bronchitis. Its diuretic and emollient qualities adapt it to urinary complaints and, as there is no astringent action (indeed, there appears to be some relaxing effect) it is particularly suitable in the treatment of nephritis, cystitis and gravel.

The powdered or crushed fresh roots make a first-rate poultice, and the leaves also are used as a fomentation in inflammation. The addition of Slippery Elm powder mproves the poultice, and the two remedies are frequently made up into an ointment for skin diseases, boils and ulcers.

The leaves are taken as an infusion of 1 ounce to 1 pint of boiling water frequently, in wineglass doses.

Culpeper relates a personal story about this herb : "You may remember that not long since there was a raging disease called the bloody flux ; the College of Physicians not knowing what to make of it, called it The Plague in the Guts, for there wits were at *ne plus ultra* about it. My son was taken with the same disease ; myself being in the country, was sent for ; the only thing I gave him was Mallow bruised and boiled both in milk and drink ; in two days it cured him, and I have here to shew my thankfulness to God in communicating it to his creatures, leaving it to posterity."

MEADOWSWEET. *Spiræa ulmaria.* N.O. *Rosaceæ.*

Synonym : Bridewort, Dolloft, Queen-of-the-Meadow.

Habitat : Low-lying meadows, sides of ditches.

Features : Stem strong, woody, reddish hue, three or four feet high. Leaves in large and small pairs, alternate, serrate ; end leaf has three leaflets with longer one in middle ; dark green on top surface, white and downy underneath. Flowers small, creamy white, clustered in large, dense cymes.

Part used : Herb.

Action : Astringent, diuretic, aromatic, tonic.

The 1 ounce to 1 pint infusion is taken in wineglassful doses for strangury and dropsy. It is especially useful in infantile diarrhœa.

Meadowsweet is included in recipes for many herb beers, its pleasantly aromatic, tonic and diuretic qualities making it particularly suitable for this purpose.

MELILOT. *Melilotus officinalis.* N.O. *Leguminosæ.*

Synonym : King's Clover.

Habitat : Waste places.

Features : Stem erect, two or three feet high. Leaves in threes, ovate-truncate, serrate, two horns at base of leaf stalk. Flowers small, yellow, in one-sided clusters. Hay-like taste and scent.

Part used : Herb.

Action : Carminative, emollient.

The 1 ounce to 1 pint infusion in wineglass doses as needed, to relieve flatulence. Sometimes used in fomentations and poultices.

MISTLETOE. *Viscum album.* N.O. *Loranthaceæ.*

Synonym : European Mistletoe, Birdlime Mistletoe.

Habitat : Parasitic on the Oak, Hawthorn, Apple and many other trees.

Features : This familiar evergreen is a true parasite, receiving no nourishment from the soil, nor even from the decaying bark. The leaves are obtuse lance-shaped, broader towards the end, sessile, and grow from a smooth-jointed stem about a foot high. The flower-heads are yellowish and the berries white. The plant is tasteless and without odour.

Part used : Leaves.

Action : Highly valued as a nervine and antispasmodic.

Mistletoe leaves are given in hysteria, epilepsy, chorea and other diseases of the nervous system. As an antispasmodic and tonic it is used in cardiac dropsy.

Culpeper is at his most "Culpeperish" in discussing this plant, as witness : "The birdlime doth mollify hard knots, tumours and imposthumes, ripeneth and discuteth them ; and draweth thick as well as thin humours from remote parts of the body, digesting and separating them. And being mixed with equal parts of resin and wax, doth mollify the hardness of the spleen, and healeth old ulcers and sores. Being mixed with Sandarack and Orpiment, it helpeth to draw off foul nails ; and if quicklime and wine lees be added thereunto it worketh the stronger. Both the leaves and berries of Mistletoe do heat and dry, and are of subtle parts."

While some truth may be hidden behind all this quaint terminology, it is feared that the modern herbal consultant would encounter serious difficulties if he attempted to follow the Culpeperian procedure too literally—although certain people still believe, or affect to believe, that he does so !

The birdlime mentioned in the quotation and also in the synonyms is the resin viscin, from the Latin *viscum*, birdlime.

MOUNTAIN FLAX. *Linum cartharticum.* N.O. *Linaceæ.*

Synonym : Purging Flax.

Habitat : Heaths, moorlands ; occasionally meadows and pastures.

Features : Stem simple, up to eight inches high. Leaves opposite, small, lower obovate, higher lanceolate, entire. Flowers small, white (June to September), five-parted with serrate sepals, pointed petals. Taste, bitter and acrid.

Part used : Herb.

Action : Laxative, cathartic.

In constipation, action similar to Senna, and sometimes preferred to the latter ; rarely gripes. Occasionally prescribed with diuretics, etc., for gravel and dropsy. Combined with tonics and stomachics such as Gentian and Calumba root, makes a first-rate family medicine. Dose, wineglass of the ounce to pint infusion.

MOUSEEAR. *Hieracium pilosella.* N.O. *Compositæ.*

Synonym : Hawkweed, Pilosella.

Habitat : Banks and dry pastures.

Features : Stem 6-8 inches, creeping, slightly hairy. Leaves form small rosettes around stem, elongate-lanceolate, hairy; given common name owing to imagined resemblance to a mouse's ear in form. Flowers lemon-coloured, outer petals tinted red underneath.

Part used : Herb.

Action : Astringent, expectorant.

The ounce to pint infusion, taken in wineglass doses, makes quite a useful medicine for whooping and other coughs.

MUGWORT. *Artemisia vulgaris.* N.O. *Compositæ.*

Synonym : Felon Herb.

Habitat : Hedgerows and about walls.

Features : Stem up to four feet, angular, longitudinal channels. Leaves alternate, five to seven lobes, silvery-white down beneath, nearly smooth above. Flowers (July and August) ovoid, purplish, in clusters. Odour aromatic, leaves slightly bitter.

Part used : Leaves.

Action : Emmenagogue, diuretic, diaphoretic.

In menstrual obstruction, usually with Pennyroyal and Southernwood. Infusion of 1 ounce to 1 pint boiling water, wineglass doses.

MULLEIN. *Verbascum thapsus.* N.O. *Scrophulariaceæ.*

Synonym : Great Mullein, Blanket Herb, or Candle Flower.

Habitat : Flourishes in sandy and gravelly waste ground, and is sometimes noticed under garden cultivation.

Features : Reaching a height of four feet, the thick, erect, un-branched stem is heavily coated with hairs. The large, flannel-like leaves are lanceolate-oblong below, the upper ones becoming decurrent, smaller, and more ovate in shape. Characteristic of the plant, leaves narrow at the base into two wings which pass down the stem, this feature enabling the medicinal Mullein to be distinguished from *Verbascum nigrum* and various other Mulleins. The flowers, which bloom in

July and August, are built of five golden-yellow, rounded petals, and are densely packed on a woolly spike some foot or more in length.

Part used : Leaves and flowers.

Action : Demulcent, pectoral and astringent.

A medicine is made by infusing 1 ounce in 1 pint of boiling water, the usual dose being a wineglassful, taken frequently. This is recommended mainly for chest coughs and certain other pulmonary complaints. Mullein has been considered a pile cure for several hundred years, and is still used for this purpose both internally and as a fomentation.

Culpeper preferred the root to the leaves and flowers, and advised it to be taken in wine. He tells us that this "is commended by Dioscorides against lasks and fluxes of the belly."

OATS. *Avena sativa.* N.O. *Graminaceæ.*

Synonym : Groats.

Habitat : Under field cultivation.

Features : Oats of commerce and general use are the seeds of *Avena sativa* with the husk removed. The crushed or coarsely powdered oats is known as groats, and the powder, either fine or coarse, as oatmeal.

Part used : Seeds.

Action : Nervine, tonic, stimulant, antispasmodic.

As a restorative in nervous exhaustion, and of particular value in correcting spasmodic conditions of bladder and ureter. Curative properties of oats may be utilized through the medium of the fluid extract. Dose, 10-30 drops.

ORRIS. *Iris florentina.* N.O. *Iridaceæ.*

Synonym : Florentine Orris.

Habitat : Cultivated in Northern Italy and Morocco.

Features : The white Florentine root, which is preferred to other varieties, is irregular in shape and shows marks where the rootlets branched before preparation for export. Verona Orris root tapers more gradually than that from Florence, and appears more compressed. The Moroccan root is noticeable for the dirty white cortex which remains on the root. Orris gives off a violet-like scent.

Part used : Root.

Large quantities of the finely pulverised root are used in the preparation of toilet and dusting powders, dentifrices and cachous, for which purposes the acceptable fragrancy and other appropriate qualities make Orris root eminently suitable. Toilet recipes are given in another section of this book.

Orris is not used for purely medicinal purposes.

OX-EYE DAISY. *Chrysanthemum leucanthemum.* N.O. *Compositæ.*

Synonym : Field Daisy, Great Ox-Eye, Horsegowan, Marguerite, Moon Daisy.

Habitat : Fields, especially near the sea.

Features : Stem from one to two feet, smooth, hard, angular, slightly branched. Leaves from lower part stalked, spatulate, serrate ; remainder sessile, serrate, oblong. Flowers large, white, daisy-like, each on its own long flower stalk.

Part used : Herb.

Action : Antispasmodic, tonic.

To some extent in whooping cough and asthma. The tonic effect is similar to that of Chamomile, but the greater popularity of the latter is probably justified. A decoction of 1 ounce to 1 pint (reduced from 1½ pints) is taken in wineglass doses, and may also be used externally for wounds and ulcers, and as an injection in leucorrhœa. Large internal doses induce vomiting.

PARSLEY PIERT. *Alchemilla arvensis.* N.O. *Rosaceæ.*

Synonym : Parsley Breakstone.
Habitat : Hedgerows, in better soils.
Features : Up to six inches in height, the whole plant rather hairy. Leaves small, trifid higher up the stem, palmate lower down. Axillary tufts of small, greenish flowers.
Part used : Herb.
Action : Diuretic, demulcent.

A widely-used diuretic acting directly on the parts. The 1 ounce to 1 pint infusion may be given in teacupful doses thrice daily in all kidney and bladder irregularities.

PELLITORY-OF-THE-WALL. *Parietaria officinalis.* N.O. *Urticaceæ.*

Habitat : Old walls.
Features : Up to two feet high, stem reddish, brittle, angular, rather hairy. Leaves alternate, stalked, lanceolate, edges smooth, one to two inches long by half an inch to one inch broad. Numerous pink flowers (June and July), small, axillar.
Part used : Herb.
Action : Diuretic, laxative.

Gravel, suppression of urine, and other bladder and kidney disorders. Frequently prescribed in combination with Wild Carrot and Parsley Piert. Wineglass doses of the infusion of 1 ounce to 1 pint boiling water.

PENNYROYAL. *Mentha pulegium.* N.O. *Labiatæ.*

Synonym : European Pennyroyal.
Habitat : Not common as a wild plant, except on damp heaths and commons. Frequently seen in cottage gardens. Indigenous to Britain and Europe.
Features : This member of the mint family grows up to twelve inches high, the stem being bluntly quadrangular. The one to one and a half inch long, egg-shaped leaves

are opposite, on short stalks; they are slightly serrate and nearly smooth. Purple flowers appear in August. The odour is rather pungent, mint-like but characteristic.

Part used : The whole herb.

Action : Carminative, emmenagogue, diaphoretic and stimulant.

An infusion of 1 ounce to 1 pint of boiling water, taken warm in teacupful doses frequently repeated, is helpful in hysteria, flatulence and sickness. For children's ailments such as feverish colds, disordered stomach and measles, Pennyroyal infusion may be given in appropriate doses with confidence. Its diaphoretic and stimulant action recommends it for chills and incipient fevers, and the infusion works as an emmenagogue when such ailments retard and obstruct menstruation. The oil of Pennyroyal is a first-rate protection against the bites of mosquitoes, gnats, and similar winged pests. The herb is used to some extent as a flavouring. Although not so popular as other herbs for this purpose, the mint-like flavour and carminative virtues of Pennyroyal should recommend it to cooks as adding to both palatability and digestibility of various dishes.

American or Mock Pennyroyal are the names given to the dried leaves and flowering tops of *Hedeoma pulegioides*. This plant, although quite different in appearance from the European Pennyroyal, has similar medicinal values.

PEONY. *Pæonia officinalis.* N.O. *Ranunculaceæ.*

Synonym : Common Peony, Piney.

Habitat : Cultivated in gardens.

Features : Stem two feet high, thick, smooth, branched leaves, pinnate or lobed. Flowers (May) large, red, single, terminal. Transverse section of root is starchy, medullary rays tinged purple. Taste sweet, becoming bitter.

Part used : Root.

Action : Tonic, antispasmodic.

Convulsive and spasmodic nervous troubles as chorea and epilepsy. Infusion of 1 ounce powdered root to 1 pint boiling water in wineglass doses three or four times daily.

PEPPERMINT. *Mentha piperita.* N.O. *Labiatæ.*

Synonym : Balm Mint, Brandy Mint.
Habitat : Damp places by water courses. Largely cultivated, especially in the U.S.A., for its oil, which is probably the most used of all the volatile oils.
Features : Stem quadrangular, purplish, reaching three or four feet high. Leaves stalked, serrate, very slightly hairy, about two and a half inches by one inch. Characteristic taste and smell.
Part used : Herb.
Action : Carminative, stomachic, stimulant.

In flatulence, colic and nausea. Usually combined with other remedies when a complete stomachic is needed. Particularly suitable for children. Dose, wineglassful of ounce to pint infusion.

PERIWINKLE. *Vinca major.* N.O. *Apocynaceæ.*

Synonym : Greater Periwinkle.
Habitat : Woods and shady banks.
Features : About a foot high, the stem is smooth and cylindrical, with the shiny egg-to-lance-shaped leaves growing opposite at intervals of two to three inches ; the larger lower leaves are one and a half to three inches long by one to two inches broad, all being entire at the edges. The bright, blue-purple, rotate flowers bloom as large as a florin. The taste is slightly bitter and acrid, and there is no smell.
Part used : The herb.
Action : Astringent and tonic.

The infusion of 1 ounce to 1 pint is useful in internal hemorrhages and diarrhœa, as a gargle for inflammatory conditions of the throat, and as an injection for menorrhagia and leucorrhœa.

Periwinkle has been employed for many years in the treatment of diabetes. A report from South Africa, stating that a registration officer in Durban was declared cured of this disease after two months treatment with the herb, aroused much attention and considerable notice in the South African and British Press. There appears to be some ground for belief that the administration of *Vinca major*, combined, of course, with proper dietetic and other treatment, can be of benefit to diabetics.

PILEWORT. *Ranunculus ficaria.* N.O. *Ranunculaceæ.*

Synonym : Lesser Celandine, Little Celandine (not to be confused with *Chelidonium majus*, q.v.).

Habitat : Moist places, both open and shady.

Features : Flower stem grows up to six inches (slightly longer than leaf stalk) with two or three leaves, and ending in a single bright yellow, buttercup-like flower, of usually eight petals and three sepals. Numerous leaves from the root on long stalks, glossy, heart-shaped, whitish-green blotches, notched margins. Root characteristically bunched into white, fleshy, club-shaped or oblong-rounded knots.

Part used : Herb.

Action : Astringent.

Used almost entirely (as the common name denotes) in the treatment of piles. The ounce to pint boiling water infusion is taken consistently in wineglass doses, and an ointment is made by macerating the herb in boiling lard for twenty-four hours. Probably the best of all known remedies for this complaint, the combination with Witch Hazel is found to be particularly effective.

PIMPERNEL, SCARLET. *Anagallis arvensis.* N.O. *Primulaceæ.*

Synonym : Poor Man's Weatherglass, Shepherd's Barometer (these names because the flowers close some hours before rain), Red Pimpernel.

Habitat : Cornfields, waste places and in gardens.

Features : Stem square, weak, much branched, trailing with tendency to ascend, between six inches and one foot long. Leaves small, opposite, ovoid, sessile, entire at edges, black dots underneath. Flowers scarlet, corolla rotate, on long, slender, axillary stalk.

Part used : Leaves.

Action : Diuretic, hepatic, diaphoretic.

The properties of this herb, although very active, are not yet fully known, and care should be exercised in using it. It has been successful in the treatment of liver irregularities, forms of rheumatism and dropsy. The pulverised leaves are administered in doses of from 15 to 60 grains.

PINKROOT. *Spigelia marilandica.* N.O. *Loganiaceæ.*

Synonym : Carolina Pink, Indian Pink, Maryland Pink, Worm-grass.

Habitat : Southern states of U.S.A.

Features : Imported root is rather less than a quarter of an inch thick, cup-shaped scars on upper surface, many rootlets underneath.

Part used : Root.

Action : Anthelmintic.

Widely used throughout the United States, where it is considered the best of the vermifuges, and is given to both children and adults suffering from the pests. A purgative such as Senna is usually added, as it is said to cause the Spigelia to act more quickly and effectively. An infusion of 1 ounce to 1 pint is given night and morning, in doses varying with the patient's age up to one teacupful for adults.

In this country such remedies as Tansy and Wormwood are more commonly prescribed in the treatment of worms.

PLANTAIN. *Plantago major.* N.O. *Plantaginaceæ.*

Synonym : Also called Ripple Grass and Waybread, the herb is known in Scotland as "Soldiers," and in America and New Zealand as "Englishman's Foot"—Plantain being supposed always to follow in his footsteps.

Habitat : Spreads in meadows, long the borders of fields, and in the hedgerows.

Features : Springing from the root, the large leaves are ovate, blunt, and contract abruptly at the base. When, however, the plant is found in open fields the leaves tend to grow upwards on channelled stalks. The very small, brownish-purple flowers grow close together on a spike about five inches long. The plant is astringent to the taste, and odourless.

Part used : The leaves are used medicinally.

Action : Alterative and diuretic.

Combined with other agents, they are of some value in piles and diarrhœa. The fresh juice will give relief from insect and nettle stings.

John Skelton writes that Plantain "makes one of the best ointments for piles I know of."

PLEURISY ROOT. *Asclepias tuberosa.* N.O. *Asclepiadaceæ.*

Synonym : Butterfly Weed, Tuber Root, Wind Root.

Habitat : Moist, loamy soil. Indigenous to U.S.A.

Features : Stem two to three feet high, contains milky juice. Root, wrinkled longitudinally, light brown outer surface, whitish internally ; fracture tough, irregular. Rootstock knotty, faintly ringed. Acrid taste.

Part used : Root.

Action : Diaphoretic, expectorant, antispasmodic.

Chest complaints ; acts directly on the lungs, and stimulates sweat glands. Relaxes capillaries, relieving strain on heart and lungs. Reduces pain and assists breathing in pleurisy. Infusion of 1 ounce of the powdered root with 1 pint of boiling water is taken in wineglass doses, to which a teaspoonful of composition powder (Myrica compound) may be added with advantage.

POKE ROOT. *Phytolacca decandra.* N.O. *Phytolaccaceæ.*

Synonym : Garget, Pigeon Berry.

Habitat : U.S.A. Cultivated on a small scale in England for medicinal purposes.

Features : The root is obtainable in longitudinally split pieces or in transverse slices. Ringed, brownish-grey externally, hard and whitish inside ; fibrous fracture. Berries purplish-black, nearly globular, ten carpels, each containing one lens-shaped seed.

Part used : Root, berries.

Action : Alterative, cathartic.

Chronic rheumatism and skin diseases. Of some use in dyspepsia. Action of root stronger than berries. For rheumatism the root is often compounded with Black Cohosh and Wintergreen.

Preparation and dosage vary considerably with the condition of the root. Thurston, Hammer and other physio-medical practitioners recommend that only the green root should be used, owing to rapid deterioration. These herbalists use the fresh root largely in hardening of the liver and reduced biliary flow.

PRICKLY ASH. *Xanthoxylum americanum.* N.O. *Rutaceæ.*

Synonym : Toothache Bush or Suterberry.

Habitat : Flourishes in moist places throughout the United States, from which country the medicinal berries and bark are imported.

Features : A shrub varying between ten and fifteen feet in height with alternate branches covered with strong, sharp prickles, the leaves are pinnate, with lanceolate leaflets, the flowers green and white. Small, blue-black berries enclosed in a grey shell grow in clusters on the top of the branches. The bark is about one-twelfth of an inch thick, and has corky, conical spines nearly one inch in height. Fractures show green in the outer part and yellow in the inner. The taste is very pungent, causing salivation, and there is little odour.

Part used : Berries and bark, the berries being considered the more effective.

Action : Stimulant, alterative, nervine and diaphoretic.

An infusion of the berries, or the crushed or powdered bark, is made in the proportion of ½ ounce to 1 pint of boiling water, the dose being one tablespoonful four times daily. The infusion should be allowed to stand in a covered vessel for two hours before use.

In the treatment of chronic rheumatic trouble this medicine is given a prominent place, and it is also widely used wherever a general stimulant is needed. The powdered bark is applied directly to indolent ulcers. As an external application for rheumatism, Coffin recommends 1 ounce of the pulverised bark to 4 ounces of Olive oil, heated, the part to be well rubbed with this liniment night and morning.

PSYLLIUM. *Plantago ovata* or *P. ispaghula, P. psyllium.*
N.O. *Plantagineæ.*

Synonym : Flea Seed, Fleawort.
Features : Over one hundred species of this genus of stemless, herbaceous plants are known to botanists. The seeds of two of these are used in herbal medicine.

Plantago ispaghula, or Light Indian Psyllium, is cultivated in India. Seeds are boat-shaped, with one end sharper than the other, and grey-brown in colour. A small brown spot is a feature of the convex side. Transparent mucilage surrounds the seeds when kept in water.

Plantago psyllium, which yeilds the so-called Dark Brilliant Indian Psyllium seeds, is indigenous to many parts of Southern Europe and Northern Africa, and is largely cultivated in France and Spain. These seeds are the most highly esteemed for therapeutic purposes, although they do not contain so much mucilage as the Ispaghula. The "English Golden" variety is even less mucilaginous, and is used mainly for feeding birds.

Psyllium seeds are tasteless and odourless, and their peculiar action on the intestines renders them of particular value in sluggishness and atony of this organ. Swelling into a demulcent, jelly-like mass, which gently lubricates and stimulates the bowels, the seeds do not gripe, and their action is certain. Probably nothing better than Psyllium seeds can be given to most people for constipation, and they are eminently suited to children. The adult dose varies between two and four teaspoonfuls after meals, children proportionately with their age.

In tropical countries the seeds are helpful in the treatment of dysentery.

PULSATILLA. *Anemone pulsatilla.* N.O. *Ranunculaceæ.*

Synonym : Easter Flower, Meadow Anemone, Pasque Flower, Passe Flower, Wind Flower.

Habitat : High pastures.

Features : Stalk up to six inches high. Leaves hairy, three to five inches long by two to three inches broad, bipinnate, leaflets opposite, stalked below. Flowers (April and May) large, single, six dull violet petals. Taste pungent when fresh.

Part used : Herb.

Action : Nervine, antispasmodic, alterative.

Nervous exhaustion in women, particularly when resulting from menstrual causes. Has a stimulating action on all mucous surfaces. Dose, 1-2 tablespoonfuls of the ½ ounce to 1 pint infusion.

PURPLE LOOSE-STRIFE. *Lythrum salicaria.* N.O. *Lythraceæ.*

Synonym : Purple Grass, Willow Strife.

Habitat : By waterways ; luxuriantly on river islands and banks.

Features : Stem four- (sometimes six-) sided, up to four feet high. Leaves in pairs, threes or fours, nearly sessile, lanceolate, margins entire, two to five inches long. Flowers (July to September) large, reddish-purple, six to eight in rings round the stalk. Root woody.

Part used : Herb.

Action : Febrifuge, astringent, alterative.

Chiefly in feverish conditions with other herbs. Sometimes as an astringent in diarrhœa. Used alone, simmer 1 ounce in 1½ pints water for ten minutes. Dose, wineglassful as required.

QUASSIA. *Picræna excelsa.* N.O. *Simarubaceæ.*

Synonym : Bitter Wood or Bitter Ash.

Habitat : A West Indian and South American tree, is imported from Jamaica, and the wood is obtainable in small, yellow chips.

Quassia wood is very commonly used as a bitter tonic and anthelmintic. Small cups known as "Bitter Cups" are sometimes made of the wood, and water standing in them soon acquires the medicinal properties of the wood. This water, or an infusion of 1 ounce of the chips in 1 pint of cold water is taken in wineglass doses as a remedy for indigestion and general debility of the digestive system. Quassia infusion is also given to children suffering from worms, in appropriate doses according to age. Midges, gnats, and other insect pests may be kept away by damping the hands and face with the liquid.

The history of Quassia wood as an agent in non-poisonous herbal medicine is interesting. The curative properties of the wood were first brought to general notice through a negro slave named Quassy, whose people in his native country of Surinam, used it as a remedy for the various fevers to which they were subject. Quassy communicated his knowledge of the tree's virtues to Daniel Rolander, a Swede, who brought specimens to Europe in 1755.

RAGWORT. *Senecio jacobæa.* N.O. *Compositæ.*

Synonym : Dog Standard, Fireweed, Ragweed, St. James's Wort, Staggerwort, Stinking Nanny.

Habitat : Pastures and waysides, especially near the sea-coast.

Features : Stem erect, striate, tough, two to three feet high. Leaves alternate, lower lyrate-pinnatifid, stalked ; upper bi-pinnatifid, sessile. Yellow flowers (July and August) florets of the ray smooth, of the disc hairy. Root consists of many long, thick fibres.

Part used : Herb.

Action : Diaphoretic, detergent, antiseptic.

In coughs, colds, influenza, catarrhs, and for the relief of sciatica and rheumatic pains, wineglass doses of the ounce to pint decoction are taken as needed. Makes a good gargle, and is applied externally to ulcers and wounds. Ragwort ointment is prepared from the fresh herb and used for inflammation of the eyes.

RASPBERRY. *Rubus idæus.* N.O. *Rosaceæ.*

Synonym : *Rubus strigosus,* American Raspberry.

Habitat : Woods and heaths ; dry, gravelly or stony ground. Also cultivated in gardens.

Features : Stem erect, freely branched, three or four feet high, covered with small, straight, slender prickles. Leaves stalked, pinnate, with two pairs of ovate leaflets and larger terminal leaflet, rounded base, doubly serrate, pale green above, grey-white down beneath, about three inches long by two inches broad. Small white, pendulous flowers (May or June) in simple clusters. Astringent to the taste.

Part used : Leaves.

Action : Astringent, stimulant.

The 1 ounce to 1 pint infusion is widely used as a mouth-wash and gargle, and for the cleansing of wounds and ulcers. Frequently combined with Slippery Elm as a poultice. With a little Ginger and Pennyroyal it is recommended for the stomach and bowel disorders of children.

Thomson and his immediate successors strongly advised

the free drinking of the Raspberry leaves infusion for several months before confinement as an aid to parturition, and it is still much in demand for this purpose.

RED CLOVER. *Trifolium pratense.* N.O. *Leguminosæ.*

Synonym : Purple Clover, Trefoil.

Habitat : Fields and roadsides.

Features : This is the common clover of the field, long cultivated by the farmer, and is found growing to a height of one foot or more. The leaves, composed of three leaflets, grow on alternate sides of the stem. The leaflets themselves are broad, oval, pointed, and frequently show a white spot. The stem is hairy and erect, and the red (or, perhaps, purplish-pink) flower-heads (the part of the plant employed in herbal practice) are formed by a large number of separate blossoms at the end of a flower stalk. Both taste and odour are agreeable.

Action : Alterative and sedative.

The infusion (1 ounce to 1 pint of boiling water, which may be drunk freely) makes a reliable medicine for bronchial and spasmodic coughs. The alterative character is best brought out in combination with such agents as Burdock and Blue Flag.

Fernie writes of Red Clover : "The likelihood is that whatever virtue the Red Clover can boast for counteracting a scrofulous disposition, and as antidotal to cancer, resides in its highly-elaborated lime, silica, and other earthy salts."

RED SAGE. *Salvia officinalis.* N.O. *Labiatæ.*

Synonym : Garden Sage.

Habitat : Cultivated in gardens.

Features : Stem and leaves reddish, grows up to about twelve inches. Stem quadrangular, slightly hairy. Leaves stalked, oblong-lanceolate, rounded at ends, crenulate at margins, reticulated both sides. Flowers labiate, reddish-purple. Taste, powerfully aromatic.

Part used : Leaves.

Action :   Aromatic, astringent, tonic, stomachic.

In the treatment of laryngitis, inflammation of throat and tonsils, and ulceration of mouth and throat. The 1 ounce to 1 pint infusion in frequent wineglass doses is given as an internal medicine, the gargle and mouth wash being made as follows : Pour ½ pint of hot malt vinegar on to 1 ounce of the Red Sage leaves, adding ½ pint of cold water.

Both Red Sage and the green-leaved variety are extensively used in the kitchen as a flavouring and digestive.

Red Sage will also tend to darken grey hair—see "Toilet Recipes."

RHUBARB, TURKEY.   *Rheum palmatum.*   N.O. *Polygonaceæ.*

Habitat :   China.
Rheum palmatum was once transported from China through Persia to Turkey and was consequently known as "Turkey Rhubarb" ; when conveyed via India it was called "East Indian Rhubarb." This Chinese root is the popular medicinal Turkey Rhubarb of to-day, the best kind being that from the Shensi province of China.

Features :   The root is smooth and heavy, and arrives in this country peeled. It is identifiable by the dark brown spots and a reticulation of white lines. The Canton rhubarb is more fibrous, unspotted, and the white network is less prominent than that from Shensi. The quality of these roots is judged by the fracture, which should show bright, the inferior kinds being a dull brown.

Action :   Aperient, stomachic, astringent, tonic.

Small doses of the powdered root are used in diarrhœa, larger quantities acting as a thorough yet gentle purgative. Dose of powdered root, 3 to 30 grains.

ST. JOHN'S WORT. *Hypericum perforatum.* N.O. *Hypericaceæ.*

Some thirteen different varieties of St. John's Wort flourish in England, but *Hypericum perforatum* is the only one included in the herbal materia medica, and may be distinguished from the others by the small hole-like dots on the leaf.

Habitat :   Hedges and woods.

Features :   The upright, woody but slender stem, branching from the upper part only, attains a height of between one and two feet. The leaves are stalkless and elliptical in shape, about half an inch long, grow in pairs on opposite sides of the stem and branches and, in addition to the transparent dots noticed above, are sometimes marked with black spots on the under side. Numerous bright yellow flowers, dotted and streaked with dark purple, cluster, in June and July, at the ends of side branches and stem. A bitter, astringent taste is remarked.

Action :   Expectorant, diuretic and astringent.

Indicated in coughs, colds, and disorders of the urinary system. It was prescribed more often by the English herbal school of a hundred years ago than it is to-day, and was noticed as far back as Culpeper for "wounds, hurts and bruises." Indeed, an infusion of the fresh flowers in Olive oil, to make the "Oil of St. John's Wort," is still used as an application to wounds, swellings, and ulcers. Internally, the infusion of 1 ounce of the herb to 1 pint of boiling water is taken in wineglass doses.

In America St. John's Wort grows freely in the cornfields, which proximity was held by Tilke to operate beneficially upon both herb and grain. Discussing American wheat which has grown among quantities of St. John's Wort he tells us : "It is well known, by almost every baker who works in his business, that this flour improves the quality of the bread, by having a small quantity of it in every batch, particularly in seasons when the English flour is of inferior quality. A clever author informs us that it contains one-fourth more gluten than our famous wheats grown in Gloucestershire, known by the name of 'rivets.' " Tilke was himself a baker in his early days.

SANICLE. *Sanicula europæa.* N.O. *Umbelliferæ.*

Synonym : Pool Root, Wood Sanicle.

Habitat : Woods and shady places.

Features : Stem nearly simple, reddish, furrowed, up to two feet high. Leaves radical, palmate, long-stalked, glossy green above, paler underneath, serrate, nearly three inches across. White, sessile flowers, blooming in June and July. Taste astringent, becoming acrid.

Part used : Herb.

Action : Astringent, alterative.

With more powerful alteratives in blood impurities. As an astringent in diarrhœa and leucorrhœa. Wineglass doses of the ounce to pint (boiling water) infusion are taken. Claims have been made for this herb in the treatment of consumption, and Skelton has given publicity to alleged cures. These cases are not now considered to have been proved.

SARSAPARILLA, JAMAICA. *Smilax ornata.* N.O. *Liliaceæ.*

Synonym : *Smilax medica, Smilax officinalis.*

Habitat : Sarsaparilla is imported from the West Indies and Mexico.

Features : The root, which is the only part used medicinally, is of a rusty-brown colour and cylindrical in shape. It is a quarter of an inch to half an inch in diameter, has many slender rootlets, is deeply furrowed longitudinally, and the transverse section shows a brown, hard bark with a porous central portion. The taste is rather acrid, and there is no smell.

The "Brown" Jamaica Sarsaparilla comes from Costa Rica. The Honduras variety reaches us in long, thin bundles with a few rootlets attached, and further supplies are imported from Mexico.

First introduced by the Spaniards in 1563 as a specific for syphilis, this claim has long been disproved, although the root undoubtedly possesses active alterative principles. It is consequently now held in high regard as a blood purifier, and is usually administered with other alteratives, notably Burdock.

Compound decoctions of Sarsaparilla are very popular as a springtime medicine, and Coffin's prescription will be found in the Herbal Formulæ section of this volume.

SASSAFRAS. *Sassafras officinale.* N.O. *Lauraceæ.*

Synonym : Kuntze.

Habitat : West Indies—imported from U.S.A.

Features : Rootbark is a bright, rusty brown, soft and brittle. Short, corky, layered fracture, with many oil cells. Chips of the woody root are commonly used—they are brownish-white in colour, showing concentric rings and slender medullary rays.

Part used : Root, bark of root.

Action : Stimulant, diaphoretic (according to Coffin mildly antiseptic and detergent also).

Combined with alteratives for the treatment of skin eruptions and uric and other acid complaints. A decoction of 1 ounce to 1 pint (reduced) is taken in frequent wineglass doses. The decoction is sometimes used externally for ophthalmia.

Powdered Sassafras root was formerly (and in some places still is) sold as a substitute for tea or coffee, under the name of salap or saloop.

SCULLCAP. *Scutellaria lateriflora.* N.O. *Labiatæ.*

Synonym : Sometimes named Skullcap, and locally known as Madweed.

Habitat : Indigenous to the United States, the plant is also found in England on the banks of streams and in wet ditches.

Features : A strong, straight, square stem reaches eighteen inches in height, and heart- or lance-shaped, tooth-edged leaves grow opposite each other on a short stalk. The pale blue flowers, with a helmet-shaped upper lip, bloom in pairs just above the leaves. Both taste and odour are feeble.

Part used : The whole herb.

Action : One of the finest nervines known to herbalism, the whole herb is also antispasmodic and tonic in action.

The properties of Scullcap are said to have been first appreciated by Vandesveer in 1772 for use against hydrophobia. Scullcap is now employed, often with Valerian, in hysteria and insomnia, and is reputed to be effective in the treatment of epilepsy.

Coffin prescribed Scullcap in powder, decoction, and infusion, his dose of the powder being from one-half to a teaspoonful. Half a teacupful of the boiling water infusion of 1 ounce to 1 pint may be taken three or four times daily. This herb deteriorates rapidly from age and heat, and it should be kept in airtight containers.

SCURVYGRASS. *Cochlearia officinalis.* N.O. *Cruciferæ.*

Synonym : Known in some parts as Spoonwort.

Habitat : Grows freely along the sea shore.

Features : The smooth, shiny stem is angular and much branched, with ovate leaves which become sessile upwards; further roundish, kidney-shaped, stalked leaves grow from the roots. Clusters of white, cruciform flowers bloom in May. The taste is pungent and cress-like.

Scurvygrass is a powerful antiscorbutic, but, as scurvy, like other "deficiency" diseases, is now prevented and cured by purely dietetic methods, the herb is but rarely used. It is, however, given a place here both for its historic interest and for the striking way in which it exemplifies the curative potency of non-poisonous herbs.

The Medical Research Council, in its publication *Vitamins : A Survey of Present Knowledge,* says :

"Scurvygrass (*Cochlearia officinalis*) . . . figures largely in old records of scurvy cures among mariners. Thus Bachstron in 1734 tells the following story : 'A sailor in the Greenland ships was so over-run and disabled with scurvy that his companions put him into a boat and sent him on shore, leaving him there to perish without the least expectation of recovery. The poor wretch had quite lost the use of his limbs ; he could only crawl about the ground. This he found covered with a plant which he, continually grazing like a beast of the field, plucked up with his teeth. In a short time he was by this means perfectly recovered, and upon his returning home it was found to be the herb scurvy grass.' (Rendering given by Lind [1757, p. 395].)."

When a well-authenticated case such as this is quoted by such a body as the Medical Research Council it should not be difficult to believe that other agents used in the herbal practice may be equally effective in illnesses not at present included in the official list of "deficiency diseases."

SEA LAVENDER. *Statice limonium.* N.O. *Plumbaginaceæ.*

Synonym : Marsh Rosemary.

Habitat : Marshes near the sea.

Features : Angular stem, nine or ten inches in height. Leaves broadly oblong, tapering to a peculiar tip, grow from the root round the flower stalk. Flowers blue, five delicate petals, clustering on branched stalks. No scent, in spite of name. Root purplish-brown, rough, spindle-shaped.

Part used : Root.

Action : Astringent.

Decoction of the powdered root (1 ounce to 1½ pints of water simmered to 1 pint) administered in wineglass doses wherever an astringent tonic is indicated. Makes an excellent gargle and mouth-wash for inflammatory conditions, and is used in certain urinary, uterine and vaginal discharges.

SELF-HEAL. *Prunella vulgaris.* N.O. *Labiatæ.*

Synonym : Heal All.

Habitat : Pastures and wastes.

Features : Stem square, smooth, up to a foot high. Leaves in pairs, one pair one side of stem, next pair opposite side ; short-stalked, slightly hairy on top side, entire at edges, broad based tapering to point, about one inch long by half-inch across. Flowers small, purplish-blue, upper lip upright, lower lip jagged, bloom in dense terminal bunch at end of stem.

Part used : Herb.

Action : Astringent.

The 1 ounce to 1 pint infusion is taken in wineglass doses for internal bleeding, used blood-warm as an injection in leucorrhœa, and may be used to gargle sore and relaxed throats.

SENNA. *Cassia acutifolia.* N.O. *Leguminosæ.*

Synonym : Alexandrian Senna, Cassia, East Indian Senna, Tinnevelly Senna.

Habitat : Imported from Alexandria, East Indies, and the Near East.

Features : Leaves, grey-green, lanceolate, unequal and varying at the base, between half an inch and one and a half inches long, and about a third of an inch across. Tinnevelly Senna leaves are broader near the middle and proportionately longer than the Alexandrian leaves. The commercial "Mecca Senna" is usually badly picked, and of poor quality generally. Pods (Alexandrian) green, about two inches by a quarter-inch ; East Indian narrower and darker coloured. Taste, sickly sweet.

Part used : Leaves, pods.

Action : Laxative, cathartic.

For occasional and chronic constipation, dyspepsia, and disordered stomach. Two ounces of the leaves may be infused in 1 pint of boiling water and allowed to stand for an hour before use in wineglass doses. Any possibility of griping will be avoided if 1 drachm of Ginger is added to the Senna leaves before infusing.

The Alexandrian leaves and pods are considered superior to the East Indian kind as, with most people, they act more mildly, but with equal certainty.

SHEPHERD'S PURSE. *Capsella bursa-pastoris.* N.O. *Cruciferæ.*

Synonym : Mother's Heart, Pickpocket, Shepherd's Sprout.

Habitat : Hedgerows, meadows, waysides, waste places.

Features : Stem erect, slightly branched, varies from a few inches to over a foot in height with the richness of the soil. Leaves irregular-lanceolate, also differing largely in size and shape with the plant's environment. Identifiable by the triangular seed vessels, thought to resemble in shape the purses of olden days. Blossoms during most of the year ; flowers very small, white, short-stalked. Odour unpleasant.

Part used : Herb.

Action : Diuretic, stimulant.

The infusion of 1 ounce to 1 pint is administered in wineglass doses for kidney complaints and dropsy. Often combined with Pellitory-of-the-Wall and Juniper berries.

SLIPPERY ELM. *Ulmus fulva.* N.O. *Urticaceæ.*

Synonym : Moose Elm, Red Elm.

Habitat : North America, particularly Canada.

Features : The dried inner bark of *Ulmus fulva* is one of the most valued articles in herbal medicine. It is tough and fibrous, becoming soft and mucilaginous when moistened. It is this mucilaginous quality which originated the popular name of Slippery Elm. The inner bark has a slight pinkish or rusty tint, is faintly striated longitudinally, has a strong characteristic odour, and the distinctive "slimy" taste.

Action : Emollient, demulcent, pectoral.

The finely powdered bark, prepared as an ordinary gruel, has shown remarkable results as a demulcent in catarrhal affections of the whole digestive and urinary tracts, and in all diseases involving inflammation of the mucous membranes. Both bronchitis and gastritis yield to its soothing and healing properties, and as a nutrient in general debility it is probably unrivalled.

A teaspoonful of the powder to 1 pint of boiling water makes the food or gruel. The powder should be first thoroughly mixed with an equal quantity of brown sugar and the boiling water added in small quantities, say four to the pint, mixing each time until a smooth result is obtained.

Slippery Elm bark coarsely powdered makes one of the best possible poultices for boils, carbuncles, chilblains, and skin eruptions generally. It soothes the part, disperses inflammation, draws out impurities, and heals rapidly.

SOAPWORT. *Saponaria officinalis.* N.O. *Caryophyll-aceæ.*

Synonym : Bouncing Bet, Bruise—wort, Fuller's Herb, Soaproot.

Habitat : Roadsides and waste places near habitations.

Features : Stem two feet high, smooth, round, thick. Leaves stalked, ovoid, two to three inches long. Flowers (August) flesh-coloured to white, five cordate petals, clustered towards end of stem.

Part used : Leaves, root.

Action : Alterative, detergent.

Skin diseases generally. Decoction of 1 ounce to $1\frac{1}{2}$ pints water simmered to 1 pint is taken in wineglass doses three or four times daily. Pronounced "soapy" properties will remove grease.

SOLOMON'S SEAL. *Polygonatum officinalis.* N.O. *Liliaceæ.*

Habitat : Rocky woods in high situations.

Features : Stem from twelve to eighteen inches high, with alternate sessile leaves. White flowers in May and June, usually solitary, stalks axillary ; black berries. Rhizome cylindrical, about half an inch diameter, transverse ridges, slightly flattened above, circular stem scars at intervals. Fracture short, yellowish, waxy. Taste mucilaginous, sweet then acrid.

Part used : Rhizome.

Action : Astringent, demulcent.

Lung complaints, when combined with other remedies. Also in leucorrhœa. Powdered root used as poultice for inflammations.

Infusion of 1 ounce to 1 pint boiling water—wineglass doses.

SOUTHERNWOOD. *Artemisia abrotanum.* N.O. *Compositæ.*

Synonym : Old Man, Lad's Love.

Habitat : The plant is frequently seen in gardens, where it is cultivated for its delicate, graceful appearance and pleasant, characteristic scent. It also grows wild on sandy heaths.

Features : Two feet stems are at first prostrate, but become erect after producing, in August, small yellow flowers in terminal leafy clusters. The greyish-green, very slender leaves, are divided into many linear segments.

Action : Emmenagogue, stimulant, antiseptic and detergent.

Southernwood is mainly employed in menstrual obstruction, frequently in combination with Mugwort and Pennyroyal. Wineglass doses are taken of the infusion of 1 ounce of the herb to 1 pint of boiling water. The powdered herb is sometimes given in teaspoonful or smaller doses to children suffering from worms, but such agents as Tansy and Wormwood are perhaps more effective as anthelmintics.

SPEEDWELL. *Veronica officinalis.* N.O. *Scrophulari-aceæ.*

Synonym : Bird's Eye, Cat's Eye, Common Speedwell, Fluellin (in Wales).

Habitat : Dry banks and sandy commons.

Features : Stem slender, creeping, covered with short hairs. Leaves opposite, oval, hairy, serrate, short-stalked, about half an inch long by a quarter of an inch broad. Flowers small, pink turning blue, in axillary spikes. Astringent to the taste, odour when dry rather tea-like.

Part used : Herb.

Action : Mildly alterative, expectorant, diuretic.

Helpful in minor skin blemishes, coughs and catarrhs. Made as tea, it resembles certain varieties of China tea, both in taste and aroma.

Tilke recommends the substitution of Speedwell and Wood Betony for tea as, in addition to their positive virtues, they produce none of the bad effects of the last-named beverage.

SPIKENARD. *Aralia racemosa.* N.O. *Araliaceæ.*

Synonym : Indian Spikenard, Pettymorrel, Spignet.

Habitat : U.S.A.

Features : Rhizome is about one inch in diameter, oblique, with concave stem scars. Root is a similar thickness at the base, wrinkled, light brown. Fracture short and whitish. Taste and odour aromatic.

Part used : Root, rhizome.

Action : Alterative, diaphoretic.

The strong alterative properties are made considerable use of in rheumatic and general uric acid disorders, as well as various skin diseases. Decoction of ½ ounce to 1½ pints (reduced to 1 pint) is taken in tablespoonful doses four times daily.

SQUILL. *Urginea scilla.* N.O. *Liliaceæ.*

Synonym : Scilla.

Habitat : Grown near the sea coast in Sicily and Malta.

Features : A large bulbous plant, Scilla is imported in the form of dried, curved segments of the white, bulbous root, which are tough, dirty white in colour, and approximate two inches long by a quarter-inch wide. The fracture is short, taste acrid. The powdered bulb is very hydroscopic, and should consequently be kept airtight. An Indian variety is used throughout the East, and has similar properties to the above.

Part used : Bulb.

Action : Expectorant, emetic.

As an expectorant for coughs and all bronchial affections. Is used generally to allay irritation of mucous surfaces. Dose, 2 to 10 grains of the powdered bulb. Large doses produce emesis.

SUNDEW. *Drosera rotundifolia.* N.O. *Droseraceæ.*

Synonym : Dewplant, Flytrap, Round-leaved Sundew.

Habitat : Bogs and marshy ground.

Features : Stem is the slender, wiry, leafless flower-stalk, about four inches high. Leaves radical, reddish, spherical, with glands exuding a sticky juice which is not dried by the sun's heat—hence the plant's common name. Flowers small, white, on one side of the flower-stalk.

Part used : Herb.

Action : Expectorant, pectoral, demulcent, antispasmodic.

Particularly in dry, tickling coughs, on which the herb seems to have almost a specific action. Of definite value in whooping-cough. The ½ ounce to 1 pint boiling water infusion is given in tablespoonful doses as required.

TANSY. *Tanacetum vulgare.* N.O. *Compositæ.*

Habitat : This common English wild plant was formerly cultivated in gardens, but is now rarely seen away from the borders of fields and waysides.

Features : The tough, slightly ribbed stems reach a height of two or three feet, terminating in the peculiar bunch of yellow, flat, button-like flowers by which the plant may be easily recognised in July and August ; the flowers look, indeed, as if all the petals had been pulled off, leaving only the central florets. Leaf stalks grow on alternate sides of the stem, the leaves themselves being six to eight inches long by about four inches broad, deeply cut pinnately. The crushed leaves and flowers give a pronounced aromatic smell, and have a bitter taste.

Tansy herb is probably the best of all the media for getting rid of worms in children, and a dose according to age should be given night and morning fasting. The infusion of 1 ounce to 1 pint of boiling water is used. The medicine is also esteemed in some quarters for the treatment of hysteria and certain other of the nervous disorders of women. For this purpose a wineglassful of the infusion should be taken frequently.

The old-time herbalists used Tansy as a stimulating tonic for a poor digestive apparatus, but to-day herbal compounds of greater efficacy are prescribed for dyspepsia.

TOAD FLAX. *Linaria vulgaris.* N.O. *Scrophulariaceæ.*

Synonym : Butter and Eggs, Flaxweed, Pennywort. The name "Toad Flax" because of a supposed similarity between the mouth of the flower and that of the toad.

Habitat : Hedgerows and cornfields.

Features : Stem one to two feet high, upright, only slightly branched. Leaves numerous, grass-like, tapering to a point. Stem and leaves are smooth, with a pale bluish hue. Flowers shaped like the snapdragon (antirrhinum), pale yellow, mouth closed by projecting orange-coloured lower lip ; clustered together at top of stem.

Part used : Herb.

Action : Hepatic, alterative, astringent, detergent.

To some extent in prescriptions for jaundice, hepatic torpor and skin diseases. Is also sometimes included in pile ointments. The 1 ounce to 1 pint infusion is taken in doses of 2 fl. ounces.

TORMENTIL. *Potentilla tormentilla.* N.O. *Rosaceæ.*

Synonym : Septfoil (seven leaf), Tormentilla.

Habitat : Dry pasture and moorland.

Features : The height of this freely-forked plant varies between six and twelve inches. The ternate, jagged-toothed leaves are rather long and narrow, the leaflets oblong in form. Upper leaves derive directly from the stem and seem to circle round it, the lower ones being frequently stalked. Flowering in June and July, the bright yellow petals are distinctly separate, and, seen from above, form an almost perfect Maltese cross. The root is brown, hard and cylindrical, with roundish swellings and tiny, thread-like rootlets. The fracture shows light brownish-red, with a large pith.

Part used : Root and herb.

Action : Tonic and astringent.

The root is regarded as one of the best and most powerful of all the herbal astringents. The decoction of 1 ounce to 1 pint (reduced) of water in wineglass doses is consequently used in diarrhœa and as a gargle for relaxed throats. It may also be used with benefit as a lotion for application to ulcers.

Tormentil was appreciated as a medicine far back in the days of Culpeper, who made his usual picturesquely extravagant claims for the herb.

VALERIAN. *Valeriana officinalis.* N.O. *Valerianaceæ.*

Synonym : Capon's Tail, Great Wild Valerian.

Habitat : Found in many damp places such as low-lying meadows and woods, about the banks of rivers and lakes, and in marshy, swampy ground generally.

Features : A handsome plant, growing from two to four feet and more high, whose stalks are round, thick, furrowed, and of a pale greenish colour. The leaves are pinnate with lance-shaped leaflets, growing opposite each other from the stem. The pink-white flowers (June to August) blossom in large tufts at the stalk head. A sweetish, disagreeable taste and unpleasant characteristic odour are given from the short, thick, greyish, many-fibred rootstock, which is the part used medicinally.

Action : Nervine and antispasmodic.

Valerian promotes sleep and is much valued in hysteria, neuralgia and nervous debility, especially when combined with Scullcap, Mistletoe and Vervain. An infusion of 1 ounce to 1 pint of boiling water is taken in wineglass doses three or four times daily. Larger doses should not be taken.

VERVAIN. *Verbena officinalis.* N.O. *Verbenaceæ.*

Synonym : *Verbena hastata.*

Habitat : Waste places and on roadsides, particularly near buildings.

Features : The tough, wiry, quadrangular, many-branched stem averages eighteen inches high. Roughish, pinnately-lobed, serrate leaves grow distantly and opposite in pairs ; the upper ones clasp the stem, while the lower ones are stalked. Small, light lilac-coloured flowers bloom in May, along thin, wiry spikes. Very bitter in taste, a slightly aromatic odour is given off when rubbed.

Action : Nervine, tonic, emetic and sudorific.

The herb was held in high repute by those who brought the Thomsonian system to this country. Coffin, writing ninety years ago, says : "As an emetic it ranks next to lobelia ; it is also one of the strongest sweating medicines in nature. It is good for colds, coughs and pain in the head, and some years ago was highly esteemed as a remedy for consumption. As an emetic it supersedes the use of *antimony* and *ipecacuanha*, to both of which it is superior, since it not only produces all the good effects ascribed to the others, but it operates without any of the dangerous consequences that ever attend the use of antimonial preparations, and cramps, and even death have been known to follow their use. . . . Vervain will relieve and cure those complaints in children which generally accompany teething ; it likewise destroys worms. Administered as a tea, it powerfully assists the pains of labour ; as a diuretic it increases the urinary discharge."

The ounce to pint infusion is now used, and taken in wineglass doses. As a nervine, Scullcap and Valerian are usually added.

VIOLET. *Viola odorata.* N.O. *Violaceæ.*

Habitat : Damp woods and other shady places.

Features : This is, perhaps, best known of all wild plants, **with** its long-stalked, heart-shaped leaves, and **delicate,** characteristically-scented and coloured flowers.

Part used : Leaves and flowers.

Action : Antiseptic and expectorant.

Remarkable claims have been made for violet leaves in the treatment of malignant tumours. The case of Lady Margaret Marsham, of Maidstone, was reported in the *Daily Mail* for November 14th, 1901. This lady, suffering from cancer of the throat, used an infusion, which was left to stand for twelve hours, of a handful of fresh violet leaves to a pint of boiling water. After a fortnight of warm fomentations with this liquid the growth was said to have disappeared.

The same newspaper, under date March 18th, 1905, told its readers that violet leaves as a cure for cancer were advocated in the current issue of the *Lancet*, where a remarkable case was reported by Dr. William Gordon, M.D. Such accounts as these, although interesting, should be read with considerable reserve.

WATER DOCK. *Rumex aquaticus.* N.O. *Polygonaceæ.*

Synonym : Bloodwort, Red Dock.

Habitat : In, or very near, waterways, lakes, ponds, ditches, and in marshes and swampy places.

Features : The largest of all the Docks, reaching up to six or seven feet. Stem erect, thick, striated, hollow, branched. Leaves very large, some two feet in length, pale green turning to reddish-brown, broad and sharp-pointed, point turning over towards the water. Flowers (July and August) small, greenish-yellow, with white threads which become brown. Root large, reddish brown, porous bark, large pith with honey-comb-like cells.

Part used : Root.

Action : Alterative, detergent.

Of value in skin diseases and sluggish liver, in which latter case it should be given in combination with a mild laxative. The dose is 3-4 tablespoonfuls of the decoction of 1 ounce to 1 pint after simmering from 1½ pints. This may be used as a mouthwash for ulcers, etc., and the powder makes a first-rate medicinal cleanser for the teeth.

Hool highly esteems Water Dock, and says: "It operates kindly and without excitement, being slow but sure in promoting a healthy action of the depurative functions of the system." He also claims diuretic and tonic qualities for the root.

WILD CARROT. *Daucus carota.* N.O. *Umbelliferæ.*

Synonym : Bird's Nest.

Habitat : Wastes, pastures and field borders.

Features : The branched stems of one to three feet high are tough and bristly. The whole plant is hairy, and the leaves are oblong and bipinnate, with acute segments. Blossoming in June and July, the umbel of white flowers usually contains one crimson flower in the centre. The root tapers, is yellowish-white, sweetish, and faintly aromatic. Wren tells us that "in taste and odour it resembles the garden carrot, but the root is small and white, not large." Ferrier, however, says of this root, "no resemblance in taste or colour to the cultivated carrot." Our own opinion is that Wild Carrot tastes like a rather distant relative of the household carrot—which it probably is.

Part used : The whole plant.

Action : Pronouncedly diuretic in action, as well as deobstruent and stimulant.

Wild Carrot naturally, therefore, takes a prominent place in many formulæ for the treatment of dropsy, gravel, retention of urine, and bladder trouble generally. Either an infusion or decoction may be prepared in the usual proportions, and doses of 2 fl. ounces taken three or four times daily.

Culpeper comments : "Wild Carrots belong to Mercury, and therefore breaketh wind, and removeth stitches in the sides, provoketh urine and women's courses, and helpeth to break and expel the stone."

WITCH HAZEL. *Hamamelis virginiana.* N.O. *Hamamelidaceæ.*

Synonym : Spotted Alder and Snapping Hazel.

Habitat : This shrub, like the Alders and the Hazel, grows in bunches as high as eight or ten feet, and is found on high lands and the stony banks of streams.

Features : The branches are flexuous and knotty, the bark smooth and grey with brown spots. The leaves are four to five inches long and about two inches broad, obovate, feather-veined, irregularly notched at the edges, smooth above and downy underneath. Yellow flowers appear in autumn, when the leaves are falling. Taste is astringent, and smell slight and agreeable.

Part used : Bark and leaves.

Action : Astringent and tonic.

A decoction of the bark, which is more astringent than the leaves, checks external and internal hemorrhages, and this astringency, when in combination with the more specific principles of Pilewort, makes one of the most effective pile medicines known. The compound can be obtained in the form of both ointment and suppositories for external application. For varicose veins an extract of the fresh leaves and young twigs of Witch Hazel is applied on a lint bandage kept constantly moist. Both decoctions of the bark and infusions of the leaves are made in the proportion of 1 ounce to 1 pint boiling water (after simmering for ten minutes in the case of the bark decoction) and taken in wineglassful doses.

WOOD BETONY. *Stachys betonica.* N.O. *Labiatæ.*

Synonym : Bishopswort.

Habitat : Thickets, woods and shady waysides.

Features : The stem of this well-known wild plant is slender, square and hairy ; it gives off a few distant pairs of rough, oblong leaves with rounded teeth. Purplish flowers, arranged in a terminal, oval spike, bloom in July and August. The roots are white and thready. Bitter to the taste, the odour is slight and pleasant.

Part used : The whole herb.

Action : Aromatic, astringent and alterative.

It is highly recommended for biliousness, stomach cramp and colic, and as a tonic in digestive disorders generally. It is a helpful component of prescriptions in the treatment of rheumatism and blood impurities. A wineglass of the ounce to pint infusion may be taken frequently.

Tilke is interesting on Wood Betony, as his remarks show that the herb was as popular a carminative a hundred years ago as it is to-day : "This herb boiled with wine or water," he tells us, "is good for those who cannot digest their meals, or have belchings and a continual rising in their stomach."

WOOD SAGE. *Teucrium scorodonia.* N.O. *Labiatæ.*

Synonym : Garlic Sage, Wood Germander.
Habitat : Heaths, commons, woods.
Features : Very similar in appearance to the ordinary garden, or culinary sage.
Part used : Herb.
Action : Diaphoretic, astringent, emmenagogue, tonic.

In feverish colds and faulty menstruation due to chills. Wineglass doses of the 1 ounce to 1 pint infusions are taken warm. Hool tells us that Wood Sage "combined with Comfrey and Ragwort, freely influences the bladder," and that it is "an appetiser of the first order, and as a tonic will be found equal to Gentian."

WOOD SORREL. *Oxalis acetosella.* N.O. *Geraniaceæ.*

Synonym : Allelujah, Cuckoo Sorrel.
Habitat : Woods and other shady situations.
Features : Separate stem for each flower and leaf grows from root ; they are round, slender, smooth, with a pinkish hue lower down. Leaves trifoliate, slightly hairy, yellow-green above, darkish purple underneath. Flowers five-petalled, white, purple veins, one to each slender flower stalk. Taste acid, rather lemon-like.
Part used : Herb.
Action : Diuretic, refrigerant.

Wineglass doses of the 1 ounce to 1 pint boiling water infusion may be given to feverish patients whenever a cooling medicine is desirable. It is also said to work well with other diuretics in certain urinary conditions.

WOODRUFF. *Asperula odorata.* N.O. *Rubiaceæ.*

Synonym : Waldmeister Tea.
Habitat : Woods and other shady places.

Features : Stem eight inches to one foot in height, slender, smooth, four-sided, brittle. Leaves lanceolate, rather rough at the edges, in rings of, usually, eight round the stem. Flowers tubular, with flattened mouth, divided into four white, cross-shaped petals, on long, axillary stalk. The dried herb smells like new-mown hay.

Part used : Herb.

Action : Hepatic, tonic.

In faulty biliary functioning and general liver sluggishness. Tonic properties particularly applicable to the digestive apparatus. Dose, two tablespoonfuls of the 1 ounce to 1 pint boiling water infusion.

WORMWOOD. *Artemisia absinthium.* N.O. *Compositæ.*

Synonym : Ajenjo, Old Woman.

Habitat : Waste ground.

Features : Stem two feet high, whitish, silky hairs. Leaves downy, three inches long by one and a half inches broad, pinnatifid, stalked, lobes linear, obtuse. Flowers (August) pale yellow with greenish tint, small, globular, clustered in erect, leafy panicle.

Part used : Herb.

Action : Tonic, stomachic, anthelmintic.

Infusion of 1 ounce to 1 pint of boiling water, taken in wineglass doses for poor digestion and debility. A reliable remedy for worms.

YARROW. *Achillea millefolium.* N.O. *Compositæ.*

Synonym : Milfoil, Nosebleed, Thousand-leaf.

Habitat : A wayside herb, also often seen in the pasture and meadow lands of Europe and the United States.

Features : Yarrow has a rough, angular stem, and grows from twelve to eighteen inches in height. The alternate leaves are pinnatifid, clasp the stem at the base, are slightly woolly, and are cut into very fine segments. The flowers are small, white (occasionally pink or purplish), daisy-like, and bloom in dense, flattened, terminal corymbs, appearing at their best in July.

Part used : Herb.

Action :   Diaphoretic, stimulant and tonic.

The herb is extremely useful in colds and acute catarrhs of the respiratory tract generally. As it has the effect of opening the pores, thus permitting free perspiration, Yarrow is taken at the commencement of influenza and in other feverish conditions. An infusion of 1 ounce to 1 pint of boiling water is drunk warm in wineglass doses. As a very popular remedy for influenza colds it is usually combined with Elder flowers and Peppermint in equal quantities. It was sometimes prescribed by the old herbalists as a tonic in nervous debility, but there are many better herbal medicines for this condition.

YERBA SANTA. *Eriodictyon glutinosum.* N.O. *Eriodictyon californicum.*

Synonym : Bearsweed, Mountain Balm.

Habitat :   Grown in, and imported from, California.

Features : Leaves elliptic-lanceolate, serrate, about three inches by one inch, shiny above, white down underneath. Taste and odour, aromatic.

Part used : Leaves.

Action :   Expectorant, tonic.

In catarrhal affections of the respiratory organs. Often a constituent of asthma prescriptions.

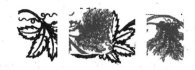

1.—INDEX TO THERAPEUTIC ACTION
of herbs comprised in the Cyclopædia

ALTERATIVES : Medicines which gradually alter and correct a poisoned condition of the blood stream and restore healthier functioning.—Blue Flag, Burdock, Celandine, Fringe-tree, Golden Seal, Plantain, Poke Root, Red Clover, Sarsaparilla, Soapwort, Spikenard, Water Dock.

ANTHELMINTICS : Remedies for worms, including those agents which kill worms (vermicides) without necessarily causing their evacuation, and those which expel them from the bowels, known as vermifuges. The term tænicide also denotes a worm destroyer.—Balmony, Pink Root, Tansy, Wormwood.

ANTISEPTICS : Resist or counteract putrefaction : Barberry, Violet, Southernwood.

ANTISPASMODICS : Reduce or prevent excessive involuntary muscular contractions.—Black Cohosh, Black Haw, Chamomile, Cowslip, Cramp Bark, Grindelia, Ladies' Slipper, Lobelia, Mistletoe, Ox-Eye Daisy, Pulsatilla, Scullcap, Sundew, Valerian.

APHRODISIACS : Tonics relating particularly to the sexual organs.—Damiana.

AROMATICS (*see* Carminatives).

ASTRINGENTS : Promote greater density and firmness of tissue, as opposed to laxatives.—Agrimony, Avens, Bayberry, Bistort, Burr Marigold, Cinquefoil, Cranesbill, Cudweed, Ground Ivy, Periwinkle, Pilewort, Red Sage, Sanicle, Witch Hazel, Wood Betony.

CARMINATIVES : Are for the dispersal of wind in stomach and bowels, and counteract griping tendencies of certain laxatives.—Angelica, Balm, Cardamoms, Catnep, Cloves, Dill, Fennel, Melilot, Peppermint, Wild Ginger.

CATHARTICS : Promote bowel evacuation, and may be divided into : (a) Laxatives, which induce gentle bowel movement ; and (b) Purgatives, producing copious, repeated, and more watery evacuations (both of which see).

DEMULCENTS : Soothe, soften and allay irritation of mucous membranes.—Blue Mallow, Bugloss, Chickweed, Comfrey, Devil's Bit, Iceland Moss, Liquorice, Marshmallow, Mullein, Slippery Elm, Solomon's Seal.

DIAPHORETICS : Induce increased perspiration.—Angelica, Balm, Boneset, Heartsease, Marigold, Pennyroyal, Prickly Ash, Ragwort, Wood Sage, Yarrow.

DIURETICS : Enhance the secretion of urine.—Broom, Buchu, Celery, Clivers, Eryngo, Gravel Root, Juniper, Parsley Piert, Pellitory-of-the-Wall, Shepherd's Purse, Wild Carrot.

EMETICS : Bring about the evacuation of stomach contents by vomiting.—Bitter Root, Lobelia, Vervain.

EMMENAGOGUES : Provoke and enhance the menstrual flow.—Black Cohosh, Mugwort, Pennyroyal, Southernwood, Wood Sage.

EMOLLIENTS : Soften, make supple, and counteract dryness and harshness of internal and external surfaces. —Liquorice, Marshmallow, Melilot, Slippery Elm.

EXPECTORANTS : Assist, by their influence on the respiratory passages, the increased secretion and ejection of mucus.—Coltsfoot, Elecampane, Horehound, Black Horehound, Lobelia, Mouse-ear, Mullein, Pleurisy Root, Squill, Sundew, Yerba Santa.

FEBRIFUGES : Reduce excessive temperature in fevers by enhancing evaporation of perspiration. Also known as refrigerants, they are closely akin to diaphoretics and sudorifics (q.v.).—Balm, Boneset, Catnep, Devil's Bit, Elder, Purple Loose-strife.

HEPATICS : Influence the liver, causing an increased flow of bile.—Chicory, Mandrake (American), Toad Flax, Woodruff.

LAXATIVES : Gently loosen the bowels.—Cascara Sagrada, Dandelion, Feverfew, Golden Seal, Mountain Flax, Psyllium, Senna, Turkey Rhubarb.

NERVINES : Relieve nervous irritation and pain.—Black Haw, Bugleweed, Mistletoe, Scullcap, Valerian.

NUTRITIVES : Assist assimilation, nourish and build tissue.—Iceland Moss, Slippery Elm.

PURGATIVES : Powerful bowel evacuatives.—Bitter Root, Bryony, Mandrake (American).

REFRIGERANTS (see Febrifuges).

SEDATIVES (see Nervines).

STIMULANTS : Produce increased nervous sensibility, with consequent improved functional action.—Adonis, Bayberry, Blood Root, Butter-bur, Cayenne, Cloves, Horseradish, Pennyroyal, Peppermint, Prickly Ash, Sassafras, Wild Ginger.

STOMACHICS : Stimulant medicines which act specifically upon the stomach.—Avens, Centaury, Chamomile, Golden Seal, Turkey Rhubarb.

SUDORIFICS (see Diaphoretics).

TÆNIFUGES (see Anthelmintics).

TONICS : Medicines which assist towards a higher bodily tone and increased vigour.—Barberry, Buckbean, Calumba, Centaury, Chamomile, Chiretta, Damiana, Gentian, Hops, Peony, Quassia, Tormentil, Vervain, Wormwood.

VERMICIDES (see Anthelmintics).

VERMIFUGES (see Anthelmintics).

2.—WEIGHTS, MEASURES & EQUIVALENTS

APOTHECARIES' MEASURE OF MASS

1 grain	= 0.0648 gramme
20 grains	= 1 scruple
3 scruples	= 1 drachm
8 drachms	= 1 ounce.

MEASURE OF CAPACITY

1 minim	= 0.0592 millilitre
60 minims	= 1 fluid drachm
8 fl. drachms	= 1 fl. ounce
20 fl. ounces	= 1 pint
8 pints	= 1 gallon

EQUIVALENTS IN DOMESTIC DOSES

1 minim	= 1 drop
1 drachm	= 1 teaspoonful
2 drachms	= 1 dessertspoonful
4 drachms (½ fl. ounce) }	= 1 tablespoonful
1½–2 fl. ounces 3–4 tablespoonfuls }	= 1 wineglassful
4–5 fl. ounces 8–10 tablespoonfuls }	= 1 teacupful

3.—MEDICINAL FORMULÆ

N.B.—These medicines ought to be made as freshly as possible—the infusions and decoctions never in quantities to last longer than four days.

An appropriate diet should be planned, and strictly adhered to, in all cases of ill-health.

Stomach and Liver

Equal parts of Golden Seal
American Mandrake
Gentian
Angelica

To 1 ounce of the mixture add 1½ pints of water, boil, and simmer to 1 pint. Wineglass doses thrice daily.

Flatulence

Balm	.	.	.	.	½ ounce
Angelica .	.	.	.	½ ,,
Pennyroyal	.	.	.	½ ,,
Cloves	.	.	.	.	1 drachm

An infusion in 1½ pints boiling water to be taken in wineglass doses (warm) as required.

Blood

Blue Flag Root	.	.	½ ounce
Burdock .	.	.	½ ,,
Red Clover	.	.	½ ,,
Yellow Dock	.	.	½ ,,
Sarsaparilla	.	.	¾ ,,
Wild Ginger	.	.	1 drachm

Boil in 3 pints of water, simmering down to 2 pints. Dose, 3 tablespoons, thrice daily.

Bronchial

Horehound	.	.	.	1 ounce
Coltsfoot	.	.	.	1 ,,
Marshmallow	.	.	.	½ ,,
Valerian .	.	.	.	½ ,,
Pleurisy Root .	.	.	½ ,,

Boil gently in 3 pints of water for 10 minutes. Dose, wineglassful three or four times daily.

Rheumatism

Equal parts of Black Cohosh
Poke Root
Prickly Ash
Agrimony
Yarrow

One ounce of the mixture to 1 pint of water, boiled, and simmered for 10 minutes. Dose, wineglassful three times daily.

Laxative (*mild*)

Dandelion Root	. .	1 ounce
Mountain Flax	. .	1 ,,
Golden Seal	. . .	1 ,,
Cloves	. . . .	½ ,,

Boil in two pints of water and simmer for 10 minutes. A wineglass to teacup dose, warm, at bedtime.

Kidney and Bladder

Buchu	. . . .	1 ounce
Parsley Piert	. . .	1 ,,
Wild Carrot	. . .	½ ,,
Pellitory	. . .	½ ,,
Juniper	. . . .	½ ,,

Decoction of 3 pints simmered to 2 pints in wineglass doses 3 or 4 times daily.

Nervine

Valerian	. . . .	1 ounce
Scullcap	. . .	1 ,,
Mistletoe	. . .	½ ,,
Wood Betony	. . .	½ ,,
Vervain	. . .	½ ,,

Boil slowly in three pints of water for 10 minutes. Dose, wineglassful thrice daily.

Composition Powder

Bayberry Bark (powdered)	1 ounce
Wild Ginger . . .	½ „
Cayenne	1 drachm

A teaspoonful of the mixture to a teacupful of boiling water is taken warm at bed-time to ward off the effects of chill, and as a general stimulant.

Coffin's Sarsaparilla Compound

"Take of sarsaparilla-root and sassafras-chips, sliced, of each one ounce ; snake-root, bruised, liquorice-root, sliced, of each half-an-ounce ; macerate them in one quart of water for ten minutes, then take out the sarsaparilla and bruise it, return it to the liquor, and boil for ten minutes ; let it stand till cool, then strain. Dose, a wineglassful three or four times a day."

4.—TOILET RECIPES

Tooth Powder

Equal parts of	Orris Root (powdered)	
	Bayberry Bark	„
	Bistort Root	„
	Prepared chalk	

To Darken Grey Hair

Grey hair may be gradually and harmlessly darkened by brushing regularly and thoroughly with the ounce to pint infusion of Red Sage. Both growth and texture also benefit.

Shampoo (General)

Balm	¼ ounce
Rosemary . . .	¼ „
Melilot	½ „
Soapwort . . .	½ „

Tie up the herbs in a linen bag and pour on them 1 gallon of boiling water. When cool enough apply all over the scalp with a cup for several minutes, massaging well with the finger-tips.

5.—CULINARY HERBS

In addition to Celery Seed, Pennyroyal and Red Sage, which have also definite medicinal purposes and are dealt with in the dictionary, the following list includes the remainder of the herbs used in the kitchen. In addition to being valuable as seasonings, their qualities as digestives make it desirable that they should be added to dishes wherever possible. The slightly medicinal action which entitles these culinary herbs to consideration as aids to digestion is shown :

Basil : Aromatic, carminative, cooling.
Bay Leaves : Carminative.
Marjoram : Tonic, stimulant.
Mint : Aromatic.
Parsley : Aperient, diuretic.
Savory : Aromatic, carminative.
Tarragon : Aromatic.
Thyme : Tonic, antiseptic.

6.—GATHERING & DRYING OF HERBS

Herbs should be gathered just after they are fully developed and are beginning to go back for the season. To dry, keeping the medicinal properties intact, they should be tied in small bunches and hung head downwards from a wire line stretched across a dry, shady and airy room. They should never be spread on the floor.

Roots should be collected only after the herb itself has fallen back for the season, no matter whether the plant is annual, biennial or perennial. Barks should never be taken from the living tree, but only in the spring time from a tree that has been cut down the previous autumn. If naturally and carefully dried, the therapeutic virtues will remain for long periods.

The above are general hints only, to which, for the expert gatherer, there will be many exceptions.

7.—GLOSSARY OF BOTANICAL TERMS

ACHENE.—A one-seeded fruit, or part of a compound fruit, seen in the Buttercup and Clematis. Does not open when ripe, and, unlike a seed, shows remnants of style or stigma at the apex.

ANTHER.—Bag containing pollen.

APPRESSED (or Adpressed).—Rising, as a leaf, parallel and close to the stem. Applied to hairs which lie close against stem, etc.

AXIL.—Angle formed by leaf or bract with stem or branch; or by branch with stem.

BIPINNATIFID.—Doubly divided in a feather-like manner.

BRACT.—An irregularly developed leaf growing from the flower stalk beneath the flower.

CALYX.—Row of floral leaves cupping the remainder of the flower.

CARPELS.—Modified leaves bearing seeds and forming the seed vessel.

CORDATE.—Heart-shaped.

COROLLA.—The inner row of floral leaves, either separate or joined together.

CORYMB.—A collective flower formation, in which the flower stalks are of differing lengths, but each rises to the same level, outer flowers being the first to open.

CRENATE.—Applied to leaves which have notched or scalloped edges.

CRENULATE.—Having very small notches or scallops at the margins.

CYME.—An inflorescence in which the central flower opens first, e.g. Elder.

DECURRENT.—Extending in a direction downward from the point of insertion.

FLEXUOUS.—Curving, winding.

FLORETS (or Flowerlets).—A little flower forming part of an aggregate one. Applied particularly to the central flowers in the flowerheads of the *Compositæ*.

GLAUCOUS.—Covered with a sea-green coloured bloom.

INVOLUCRE.—A group or ring of bracts.

LABIATE.—Applied to an irregular, monopetalous corolla.

LAMINATE.—Composed of thin layers.

LANCEOLATE.—Oval, with tapering ends.

LENTICELS.—Corky developments of the breathing pores of leaf, bark, etc.

LINEAR.—Slender.

LYRATE.—Lyre-shaped ; said of pinnatifid leaves where the terminal lobe is rounded, and larger than the others.

OBOVATE.—Inversely ovate.

OVARY.—The fruit containing seeds.

OVATE.—Egg-shaped.

OVOID.—Nearly egg-shaped.

OVULE.—An embryo seed.

PANICLE.—An inflorescence of which the first branches themselves branch, the outside flowers of each branch being the first to open.

PAPILLÆ.—Small protuberances, sometimes threadlike.

PAPPUS.—A feathery, hairy calyx.

PEDUNCLE.—Flower stalk.

PETIOLE.—Leaf stalk.

PINNATE.—Cleft in a feather-like way to the midrib.

PINNATIFID.—Divided about half-way to the midrib or rachis in a feather-like manner.

RACEME.—A form of inflorescence, as in the Currant, in which the flowers grow from a central stem, on branchlets of equal length, the lowest flower opening first.

RADICAL.—Proceeding immediately from root or rootstock.

RECURVED (or Recurvate).—Curved or bowed downward.

REVOLUTE.—Rolled back at the edges.

RHIZOME.—A more or less underground, creeping stem, which sends out shoots above and roots below.

RHOMBOID.—Shaped as a rhomb.

ROTATE.—Wheel-shaped.

SEPAL.—A division of the calyx, corresponding with "petal."

SERRATE.—Obliquely toothed as a saw.

SESSILE.—Stalkless.

SPATULATE.—Shaped as a spatula, or flattened spoon.

STAMEN.—The male organ of a flower.

STRIATE (or Striated).—Streaked with fine parallel or wavy lines.

STROBILE.—A catkin, the carpels of which are scale-like as in the pines.

STYLE.—The middle, thread-like portion of the female organ of a flower.

TERNATE.—Applied to a leaf divided into three segments.

THALLUS.—The flat, branching growth of mosses and lichens.

TRIFID.—Nearly cleft into three segments.

TRIFOLIATE.—With three distinct leaflets as Clover.

TRUNCATE.—Appearing as though cut off at the tip.

UMBEL.—An aggregate of flowers, the stalks of which all proceed from a single point and are of equal length, the outer flowers opening first.

WHORL.—An arrangement of a number of leaves or flowers around a stem, on the same level with each other.

Milton Keynes UK
Ingram Content Group UK Ltd.
UKHW041010061024
2026UKWH00002B/13